Shanghai Key Books

上海市重点图书

An English-Chinese Guide to Clinical Treatment of Common Diseases

（英汉对照）常见病临证要览

Typical TCM Therapy for Chronic Gastritis
慢性胃炎的中医特色疗法

Compiled by Guo Haiying Wang Yue

郭海英　汪悦　编著

Translated by Xie Jianqun Zheng Linyun

谢建群　郑林赟　翻译

Shanghai University of Traditional
Chinese Medicine Press

上海中医药大学出版社

图书在版编目（CIP）数据

慢性胃炎的中医特色疗法 / 郭海英，汪悦编著；谢建群，郑林赟译．—上海：上海中医药大学出版社，2004.

（（英汉对照）常见病临证要览）

ISBN 7-81010-792-5

Ⅰ．慢…　Ⅱ．①郭…②汪…③谢…④郑…
Ⅲ．慢性病：胃炎—中医治疗法—英、汉
Ⅳ. R259.733

中国版本图书馆 CIP 数据核字（2004）第 042864 号

慢性胃炎的中医特色疗法　　　　　　郭海英　汪悦　编著

上海中医药大学出版社出版发行　　　　（http://www.tcmonline.com.cn）
（上海浦东新区蔡伦路 1200 号　　　　　　邮政编码 201203）
新华书店上海发行所经销　南京展望文化发展有限公司排版　上海市印刷七厂一分厂印刷
开本 850mm×1168mm　　1/32　印张 8.875　字数 178 千字　印数 1－3100 册
版次 2004 年 9 月第 1 版　　　　　　　　　印次 2004 年 9 月第 1 次印刷

ISBN 7-81010-792-5/R·754　　　　　　　　　　定价：22.00 元
（本书如有印刷、装订问题，请寄回本社出版科，或电话 021-51322545 联系）

Compilation Board of the Guide

《(英汉对照)常见病临证要览》
编纂委员会

主　任　谢建群　吴勉华

副主任　汪　悦　丁年青

主　编　吴勉华　汪　悦

主　译　谢建群

副主编　黄桂成　王　旭

副主译　丁年青　黄国琪

编　委（按姓氏笔画为序）

田开宇	冯　丽	孙玉明	朱玉琴
朱忠宝	乐毅敏	成肇智	李七一
吴　敏	吴承玉	汪腊萍	张　琴
张传儒	沈卫星	杨亚平	杨智军
周　鲁	周　愉	周学平	郑林赟
郑耀珏	胡克武	洒荣桂	赵和庆
唐国顺	顾学兰	徐　瑶	徐小燕
陶锦文	黄月中	覃百长	薛博瑜
魏　敏			

出版人　朱邦贤

中文责任编辑（按姓氏笔画为序）

马胜英	王玲琍	王德良	何倩倩
沈春晖	单宝枝	姜水印	秦葆平
钱静庄	葛德宏		

英文责任编辑　单宝枝　姜水印　肖元春

英文特邀编辑　李照国

美术编辑　王　磊

技术编辑　徐国民

Foreword

Traditional Chinese Medicine (TCM), a great treasure of world medical science, has the history of thousands of years. It has obtained remarkable attraction and reputation in the global medical society with its new image of "nature, security, and effectiveness". More and more people over the world accept the TCM. It is our unshirkable duty, as the descendents of the Chinese doctors, to make TCM in progress so as to benefit the health of human beings.

We compiled the series of "An English-Chinese Guide to Clinical Treatment of Common Diseases" in order to assist foreign students to have a better study of clinical knowledge of TCM. The series also meet the need of Chinese doctors when they spread TCM for foreign practitioners. The series are scientifically-organized reference books which could generally reflect the updated development of clinic in TCM.

The series were written and compiled by medical professionals and English experts from 7 TCM universities or colleges including Nanjing University of TCM,

Shanghai University of TCM, Guangzhou University of TCM, etc. The faculty from Nanjing University of TCM compiled the Chinese part. Shanghai University of TCM with other colleges and universities were responsible for the translation. The proposal was drafted in 1998. After 5-year continuous adaptation, the whole series were finally completed in 2003.

The first series include ten books. They cover ten commonly-encountered diseases of viral hepatitis, primary glomerulonephritis, chronic gastritis, lung cancer, bronchial asthma, diabetes, primary hypertension, rheumatoid arthritis, cervical spondylosis, and cholelithiasis and their special treatment in traditional Chinese medicine. Each book consists of three parts. Part one discusses the major points in diagnosis and pathogenesis and pathology of the disease. Part two focuses on the typical therapy in TCM. It covers internal therapy, external therapy, acupuncture and moxibustion, Tuina (Chinese massage), physiotherapy, dietetic therapy, mental therapy, and regimen. Part three illustrates the academic experience of 3 – 4 celebrated doctors and the effective cases that they treated.

Wu Mianhua, Wang Yue, Huang Guicheng, Wang Xu and over ten professionals from Nanjing University of TCM have made great contribution. Ding Nianqing,

Huang Guoqi, Zheng Linyun from Shanghai University of TCM, Tao Jinwen from Nanjing University of TCM, Huang Yuezhong from Guangzhou University of TCM, Tian Kaiyu from Henan College of TCM, Le Yimin from Jiangxi College of TCM, Cheng Zhaozhi from Hubei College of TCM, and Tang Guoshun from Shanghai Information Institute of TCM have finished the translation through their diligent work. Professor Ou Ming from Guangzhou University of TCM, Professor Li Zhaoguo from Shanghai University of TCM and Professor Zhu Zhongbao from Henan College of TCM spent their valuable time on the proofreading and adaptation. Acknowledgement is also given to the leaders and editors from Shanghai University of TCM Press for their great support in publishing the series.

All the diseases selected in the series are frequently encountered in the clinic. The description is brief and to the point. The translation is accurate and standard. But it is not easy to precisely translate the theoretical and clinic terminology of TCM into English. Although all the members have made their great efforts, the limitation of the knowledge and different style in composition and translation will still leave the errors and mistakes. Comments and suggestions from colleagues at home and abroad are really appreciated, so that we will make improvement in

Typical TCM Therapy for Chronic Gastritis

the revised edition in future.

Xie Jianqun

Shanghai University of Traditional Chinese Medicine

December, 2003

序　言

　　数千年中华文化历史积淀铸就的中国医药学是世界医学的瑰宝,今天她正以"绿色"、"安全"、"有效"的崭新面貌,赢得了国际医学界的赞誉,也日益为世界上越来越多的国家和人民所接受。将中国传统医学进一步发扬光大,使之造福于全人类的健康,这是我辈岐黄传人义不容辞的职责。

　　为了使海外留学生能更好地学习中医的临床技能,也为了适应中国临床医师对外传播中医药学的需要,我们组织编写了这套《(英汉对照)常见病临证要览》,旨在提供一套科学规范、能全面反映中医临床诊疗实践与发展的对外交流的教学参考丛书。

　　本书由南京中医药大学、上海中医药大学、广州中医药大学等 7 所中医院校有关临床专家和英语教授合作编撰。其中,南京中医药大学负责中医临床等方面内容的编审,上海中医药大学汇合其他各院校负责英语编译。全书的编写大纲草拟于 1998 年,期间历经反复斟酌、修改,历时五载,终于 2003 年底基本定稿,可以与中医界同仁和广大读者见面了。

　　本丛书首先推出 10 册,每册分上、中、下三篇,分别介绍病毒性肝炎、原发性肾小球肾炎、慢性胃炎、肺癌、支气管哮喘、糖尿病、高血压病、类风湿关节炎、颈椎病及胆石症等

慢性胃炎的中医特色疗法

5

临床常见病的中医特色疗法。上篇为总论,概述各病种的诊断要点、病因病机;中篇专论中医对该病症的临床特色疗法,包括内治、外治、针灸、推拿、体疗、食疗、情志疗法、摄生调护等;下篇介绍了 3～4 位著名老中医的学术经验与医案。

南京中医药大学的吴勉华、汪悦、黄桂成、王旭等 10 多位专家为本书中文稿的编审付出了很多心血,上海中医药大学的丁年青、黄国琪、郑林赟,南京中医药大学的陶锦文,广州中医药大学的黄月中,河南中医学院的田开宇,江西中医学院的乐毅敏,湖北中医学院的成肇智,以及上海中医药情报研究所的唐国顺等专家为本书的译文尽心尽力;广州中医药大学欧明教授、上海中医药大学李照国教授、河南中医学院朱忠宝教授也为本书译文的润色修饰耗费了很多宝贵的时间,上海中医药大学出版社领导和编辑部的同志们为本书的出版倾注热情,大力支持,在此谨致深深的谢意。

在编写过程中,作者力求做到所选病种常见、多发,文字简明扼要,译文准确规范。然而,要把中医理论及其临床术语翻译为英语,并能准确表述其内涵,难度可想而知。尽管我们作了极大努力,囿于作者的学识,再加上撰写者行文风格的差异,粗疏之处在所难免,诚望海内外同道不吝指教,以便在今后修订时能进一步得以提高和改进。

谢建群

2003 年 12 月

于上海中医药大学

慢性胃炎的中医特色疗法

Preface

Chronic gastritis is one of the commonly encountered diseases. The incidence of this disease in adult is over 20% and increases with age. Chronic gastritis is hard to cure and tends to change into cancer, especially in the patients with gastratrophia accompanied with intestinal metaplasia or atypical hyperplasia. So it is important to prevent and treat chronic gastritis.

The history to treat chronic gastritis with traditional Chinese medicine (TCM) is long and rich experience is accumulated in this aspect. In recent years, with the development of TCM and study of this disease, more methods have been developed to treat this disease. Clinical therapeutic effect is gradually increased. This method is very popular now because it is a natural therapy with high curative effect. In order to summarize clinical experience in treating this disease, we have compiled this book based on our clinical practice and concerned literature.

This book is composed of three parts, concentrating on introduction to the treatment of chronic gastritis with traditional Chinese therapy. The first part introduces the

Typical TCM Therapy for Chronic Gastritis

concept, clinical characteristics and essentials for the diagnosis of this disease as well as its cause and pathogenesis based on TCM. The second part introduces the treatment of this disease based on syndrome differentiation, proved remedies, Chinese patent medicines, external therapies, acupuncture and moxibustion as well as dietetic therapy. The third part introduces experiences of celebrated doctors of TCM in China.

This book is characterized by rich content and concise description. It is easy to read and understand, very practical for doctors and other readers to consult in dealing with chronic gastritis.

Guo Haiying

In Nanjing University of TCM

December, 2003

前　言

　　慢性胃炎是临床常见疾病之一,成人发病率一般在20%以上,且随年龄的增长而增高。慢性胃炎日久不愈,尤其是萎缩性胃炎伴肠黏膜上皮化生或不典型增生者,有癌变的可能。因此,积极防治慢性胃炎有非常重要的意义。

　　中医学治疗慢性胃炎有悠久的历史,积累了丰富的经验。特别是近年来,随着中医学的发展,对慢性胃炎的认识更加深入,治疗方法不断扩充,临床疗效逐渐提高。作为独特的无明显毒副作用的天然疗法及其显著的疗效,用中医药方法治疗慢性胃炎越来越受到人们的欢迎。为了更好地总结中医药治疗本病的临床经验和研究成果,我们根据多年来运用中医药治疗本病的实践经验,并结合有关文献资料,编撰了此书。

　　全书共分上、中、下三篇,围绕中医治疗慢性胃炎的特色疗法进行介绍,其中上篇着重介绍慢性胃炎的概念、临床特征、诊断要点和中医学对本病病因病机的认识;中篇较详实地介绍了本病辨证治疗、单方验方、中成药、外治疗法、针灸推拿与情志、饮食疗法等;下篇则介绍了全国知名老中医一些独特的治疗经验与特色。

　　本书内容丰富,融科学性、知识性于一体,简明扼要,通俗易懂,实用性强,可供广大医务工作者和中医爱好者参考,也是慢性胃炎患者的良师益友。

由于时间仓促,编者水平有限,书中疏漏、不足之处难免,诚望广大读者不吝指教。

郭海英

2003 年 12 月

于南京中医药大学

Contents

Part One General Introduction

Part Two Characteristic Therapy

Typical TCM Therapy for Chronic Gastritis

Part Three   Experience of Famous Senior TCM Doctors

Typical TCM Therapy for Chronic Gastritis

Contents

Typical TCM Therapy for Chronic Gastritis

Contents

目　录

上篇　总　论

中篇　特　色　疗　法

慢性胃炎的中医特色疗法

下篇　名老中医治验

慢性胃炎的中医特色疗法

Typical TCM Therapy for Chronic Gastritis
慢性胃炎的中医特色疗法

Part One General Introduction

Chapter One Outline

Chronic gastritis is an inflammatory lesion of gastric mucosa layer caused by various reasons. The clinical manifestations are discomfort or pain in epigastrium, anorexia, nausea and vomiting, belching, loose stool and so on. For lack of the typical clinical symptoms, it is apt to be confused with other digestion diseases. In recent years, the wide use of gastrofiberscope is helpful for diagnosis. According to statistics, the incidence of this disease is very high. The incidence in adult is above 20%, which will be higher with getting older. For the patients who are not recovered for a long time, there are small parts of the chronic gastritis which will change to cancer, especially in atrophic gastritis. Some scholars call this disease as precancerous lesion. According to some data, among the cases of gastric cancer, there are 50%-90% of chronic atrophic gastritis and metaplasia of intestinal epithelium. In chronic gastritis, particularly in gastric antrum, the rate of canceration is high. So prevention and

上篇 总 论

一、概述

慢性胃炎是由各种原因引起的胃黏膜层的炎性病变,临床上多表现为上腹部不适或疼痛、食欲减退、恶心呕吐、嗳气、便溏等。由于本病患者缺少特异性症状,故很容易与其他消化道疾病混淆。近年来纤维胃镜在诊断中的广泛应用,对本病明确诊断有很大的帮助。据统计,本病的发病率甚高,成人的发病率一般在20%以上,且随年龄增长而增高;日久不愈的患者,有些病例可发生癌变,尤其是萎缩性胃炎,有些学者称之为癌前期疾患。据有关资料报道,胃癌病例中,50%～90%有慢性萎缩性胃炎和肠黏膜上皮化生病变;尤其是胃窦部的慢性胃炎,其癌变率更高。因此,慢性胃炎的防治越来越受到重视。

慢性胃炎的中医特色疗法

3

treatment of chronic gastritis is constantly emphasized.

According to the morphologic change of gastric mucosa under gastrofiberscope, this disease can be divided into two kinds: chronic superficial gastritis and chronic atrophic gastritis. The inflammatory change of the chronic superficial gastritis at first only involves superficial layer of gastric mucosa, but later can involve deep layer. When chronic superficial gastritis is progressing, the propria gland is decreased because of inflammatory destruction, which can transforms to atrophic gastritis. Chronic atrophic gastritis is a pathologic lesion in which the propria gland of gastric mucosa atrophy (the number decreased and function reduced) appears, usually accompanied by intestinal metaplasia and inflammatory reaction. Some scholars suggest that the chronic atrophic gastritis should be divided into two kinds: type A (inflammation of stomach body, positive of parietal cell antibody) and type B (antral gastritis, negative of parietal cell antibody).

The cause of the disease is not clear. It probably results from acute gastritis, gradual progressing from lingering gastric mucosa pathological process or the patients who take stimulating food and medicine for a long time, or over smoking and drinking, causing the lesion of gastric mucosa. On the other hand, owing to the dysfunction of sphincter muscle of pylorus, duodenal ulcer or postcholecystectomy, the bile

根据纤维胃镜下胃黏膜的形态变化,本病可分为慢性浅表性胃炎和慢性萎缩性胃炎两型。慢性浅表性胃炎最初炎性变仅累及胃黏膜的浅层,但亦可累及深层。慢性浅表性胃炎进一步发展,固有腺体因炎症破坏而减少,可以转化为萎缩性胃炎。慢性萎缩性胃炎是以胃黏膜固有腺体萎缩(数量减少,功能减低)为其突出的病变,常伴有肠上皮化生及炎性反应。有的学者主张以病变部位结合血清壁细胞抗体的检测结果作为依据,将慢性萎缩性胃炎分为 A 型(胃体炎,壁细胞抗体阳性)和 B 型(胃窦炎,壁细胞抗体阴性)。

本病的病因尚不十分明确,可能由于急性胃炎后,胃黏膜病变持续不愈演变而来,或有些患者因长期服用对胃黏膜有刺激的食物与药物,或过度吸烟与饮酒,而引起胃黏膜损害。此外,由于幽门括约肌功能失调、十二指肠溃疡或胆囊切除术后,胆汁返

regurgitates and enters into the stomach, destroying barrier of gastric mucosa, leading to the chronic gastritis. There were some reports in recent years that detectable rate of pyloric spirillum in chronic gastritis is very high. This refers to the close relationship between pyloric spirillum and inflammation of gastric mucosa.

Chapter Two   Diagnostic Main Points

Section One   Clinical manifestations

There are no clear symptoms and signs of the chronic superficial gastritis. Some patients show the manifestations of stomach upset, vague pain, anorexia, stomachache after meal, etc. If there exists regurgitation, the continuing epigastralgia, usually accompanied by reflux esophagitis, will happen. It usually has no clear signs. Sometimes there is slightly tenderness in epigastrium. The clinical manifestations of chronic atrophic gastritis show difference from pathologic degree. Some patients have no clear symptoms, but many of them have chief complaint as burning pain, dull pain, fullness (especially after meal), anorexia, nausea, and belching, etc. In serious patients, there are marasmus, iron-deficiency anemia. Some patients who have gastric mucosa erosion can have

流入胃,破坏胃黏膜屏障,而导致慢性胃炎。近年来报道幽门螺杆菌在慢性胃炎患者中检出率很高,说明其与胃黏膜炎症有密切的关系。

二、诊断要点

(一)临床表现

慢性浅表性胃炎症状与体征多不明显,部分患者有胃部不适、隐痛、嗳气、食欲不振、食后胃部疼痛加重等表现。若同时有胆汁返流存在时,常表现为持续性上腹部疼痛,亦可伴有反流性食管炎。一般无明显的体征,有时上腹部有轻度压痛。慢性萎缩性胃炎的临床表现与病变程度并不一致。有些患者可无明显症状,但大多数患者主诉上腹部灼痛、钝痛或饱胀,尤以食后为甚,以及食欲不振、恶心、嗳气等症状。严重者可有消瘦、缺铁性贫血,少数有胃黏膜糜烂者可伴上消化道出血。

慢性胃炎的中医特色疗法

7

hemorrhage of upper digestive tract.

Section Two   Physicochemical examination

1. Gastric juice analysis

The gastric acid secretion of chronic superficial gastritis usually is normal but sometimes the acidity can be low or high. In atrophic gastritis, the quantity of gastric secretion is less than that in healthy people. The degree of achlorhydia can be defined on the basis of the position and range of atrophic lesion. If the lesion is limited in gastric antrum, the gastric acid can be normal or on the low side. If it is limited in the body of stomach and the parietal cells were seriously damaged or the atrophy of most gland, hypohydrochloria or achlorhydia can happen. The quantity of basic gastric acid secretion for per hour, the largest quantity of gastric acid secretion and peak quantity of acid secretion can be assayed with the method of increasing histamine or five peptide gastrin dosage in order to know the degree of achlorhydia and pH value. If the pH value is not as low as 7.0, it is called no gastric acid; if it is as low as 3.5, it is called low acid. This can contribute to diagnosis of atrophic gastritis.

2. Gastroscopy

It is believed that gastroscopy is the most reliable method in diagnosing chronic gastritis. The lesion of

（二）理化检查

1. 胃液分析

慢性浅表性胃炎胃酸分泌一般正常，但有时酸度较低或较高。而萎缩性胃炎胃液分泌量一般较正常人为少。胃酸缺乏的程度根据萎缩病变部位和范围而定，如胃窦部病变局限，其胃酸可正常或偏低；如病变在胃体部，壁细胞损害严重或大部分腺体萎缩者，则可出现胃酸很低或无胃酸分泌。用增大组胺或五肽胃泌素剂量的方法测定每小时基础胃泌酸量、最大泌酸量和高峰泌酸量，以了解胃酸缺乏的程度，并测定 pH 值。如胃酸 pH 不低于 7.0 者，称无胃酸；如不低于 3.5 者，称为低酸，有助于萎缩性胃炎的诊断。

2. 胃镜检查

胃镜检查是诊断慢性胃炎最可靠的方法。慢性浅表性胃炎病变多

chronic superficial gastritis can be found mostly in gastric antrum. The manifestations are gastric mucosa hyperemia, edema, increasing of light reflection, red alternate with white taking red hyperemia as the dominant, or having scattered bleeding and erosion which attaches white or yellow mucus. This is usually accompanied by bile regurgitation and prolapse of gastric mucosa. The examination of histology shows the pathologic change of chronic superficial gastritis. The gastric mucosa of atrophic gastritis usually assumes pale or greyish white. The plica becomes fine or smooth. The mucosa can be marked by alternation of the red with white. Some severe cases can have scattered white spots. The exposure of blood vessel under mucosa indicates the characteristics of atrophic gastritis. Vein can be bright blue arborescent, sometimes red reticular ramular vein or capillary can be seen. In severe atrophic gastritis, microgranule or bigger node formed by epithelial hyperplasia can be seen. The phenomenon of mucosal erosion and bleeding can also be seen.

3. Pepsinogen determination

The pepsinogen is secreted by gastric cells. In chronic atrophic gastritis, the content of pepsinogen decreases in blood, and the urine can help diagnosis.

4. Gastrin determination

Determining the content of pepsinogen in blood

见于胃窦部，表现为胃黏膜充血、水肿，反光增强，红白相间，以充血的红色为主，或有散在的出血和糜烂，可有白色或黄色黏液附着。常伴有胆汁返流和胃黏膜脱垂。组织学检查呈慢性浅表性胃炎病理变化。萎缩性胃炎的胃黏膜多呈苍白或灰白色，皱襞变细或平坦。黏膜可表现红白相间，严重者有散在白色斑块。黏膜下血管显露为萎缩性胃炎的特征，呈蓝天色树枝状为静脉，有时可见到红色网状小支脉或毛细血管。严重萎缩性胃炎可见有上皮细胞增生形成细小颗粒或较大结节，亦有黏膜糜烂、出血现象。

3. 胃蛋白酶原测定

胃蛋白酶原由胃细胞分泌，慢性萎缩性胃炎时，血、尿中的胃蛋白酶原含量减少可助诊断。

4. 胃泌素测定

测定血清胃泌素含量，有助于区

serum contributes to differentiation of atrophic gastritis type A from type B. In type A, if the parietal cell antibody is positive, the blood serum gastrin in fasting clearly gets higher. In type B, if the parietal cell antibody is negative in which the gastric antrum has serious inflammation, the quantity can be normal or lower.

5. The parietal cell antibody

When there is atrophic gastritis, the serum parietal cell antibody shows positive while there is atrophic antral gastritis, the serum parietal cell antibody usually shows negative.

6. Pylorus spirillum examination

It can be tested by culture, smear and urea enzyme assay.

Section Three   Differential diagnosis

The chronic gastritis should be differentiated from gastroneurosis, ulcer and earlystage of gastric cancer. It is not difficult with the aid of gastroscope, gastric mucosa biopsy and X-ray barium meal examination of gastrointestinal tract.

别 A 型或 B 型萎缩性胃炎。A 型壁
细胞抗体阳性者,空腹血清胃泌素常
明显增高,而 B 型壁细胞抗体阴性,
胃窦部黏膜有严重炎症者,其含量可
正常或降低。

5. 壁细胞抗体

萎缩性胃体炎时,血清壁细胞抗
体常呈阳性,而萎缩性胃窦炎时则血
清壁细胞抗体多呈阴性。

6. 幽门螺杆菌检查

可通过培养、涂片、尿素酶测定
等方法检查。

(三) 鉴别诊断

本病应与胃神经官能症、溃疡病
和早期胃癌等病相鉴别,借助胃镜和
胃黏膜活检及 X 线胃肠钡餐摄片检
查,一般不难鉴别诊断。

慢性胃炎的中医特色疗法

Chapter Three   The Understanding of TCM on Chronic Gastritis

In TCM, the chronic gastritis belongs to the syndrome category of "epigastralgia", "thoracic fullness", "vomiting", "gastric upset", "acid regurgitation", etc.

The TCM believes that the chronic gastritis results from improper diet, hunger and fullness changeable, or overeating raw and cold food, stimulating food, oversmoking and drinking, which damages the spleen and stomach up to the un-descending of gastric qi, activities of qi retardation; or emotional disturbance, disorder of the liver-qi, run wild over stomach; or stagnation of the liver-qi due to fire-transmission, fire burning gastric yin; or stagnation of qi and blood stasis due to protracted disease, stomach collateral block.

1. Diet disturbance, blockage of the middle energizer

It is due to crapulence, diet disturbance, dyspeptic retention, blockage of the middle energizer; or deficiency of the spleen and stomach, dyspepsia making retention of food in stomach, injuring stomach qi which loses the function of digestion, leading to the symptoms as gastrypalgia, pantothenic acid and vomiting.

三、中医学对本病的认识

本病属于中医学"胃痛"、"痞满"、"呕吐"、"嘈杂"、"吞酸"等病证范围。

中医学认为,本病常由于饮食不节,饥饱无常,或过食生冷、刺激性食物,以及过度吸烟饮酒,损伤脾胃,以致胃失和降,气机阻滞;或因情志失调,肝失疏泄,横逆犯胃,或肝郁化火,火灼胃阴;或病久气滞血瘀,胃络阻滞等引起。

1. 饮食失节,阻滞中焦

多因暴饮暴食,饮食不节,食滞不化,阻滞中焦;或因脾胃素弱,食入难以消化,致食积胃腑,损伤胃气,胃失腐熟消化之用,而见胃脘隐隐作痛,或泛酸、呕吐等症。

2. Unsuccessful therapy, invasion of the stomach

There is acute or chronic inflammation of laryngeal part of pharynx with repeated attack, in which bacteriotoxin can directly stimulate gastric mucosa, making the stomach bradydiastalsis, the ability of digestion decreasing. Thoracic fullness and pain in the stomach, belching, acid regurgitation, vomiting and nausea, and hiccup can be seen.

3. Hyperpyrexia of stomach, deficiency of stomach-yin

There is exuberant pathogenic fire in the stomach, re-attack of febrile disease, leading to injury of the stomach-yin; or over eating hard liquor and some pungent or dryness food like chilli; or yin deficiency due to senility, deficiency of the stomach-yin, interior heat with burning stomach-yin, failure in descending of stomach-qi. Stomachache and acid regurgitation can be seen.

4. Deficiency of spleen and stomach, deficient cold in the middle energizer

The spleen and stomach is always weakness, catching cold again; or being fond of cool and drinking cool, impairing spleen and stomach; or over sprain, impairing yang-qi of the middle energizer, leading to the middle energizer cold, deficiency of yang-qi, the spleen and stomach losing warm nourish. The stomachache and anorexia

2. 治疗不利,侵及胃脘

咽喉部急性或慢性炎症,反复发作,持久不愈,细菌毒物直接刺激胃黏膜,使胃腑蠕动弛缓,腐熟能力减退,而见胃脘部痞满、疼痛,或嗳气、吞酸、呕恶、呃逆等症。

3. 胃热炽盛,胃阴亏损

胃中火热素盛,复患热性疾病,损耗胃阴;或过饮烈性白酒和过食辣椒等辛燥之物;或因老年阴亏,胃液不足,而致内热炽盛,灼伤胃阴,胃失濡降,而见胃痛、吐酸等症。

4. 脾虚胃弱,中焦虚寒

素体脾胃虚弱,复感寒邪;或夏日贪凉饮冷,损伤脾胃;或劳损过度,损伤中焦阳气,致中焦虚寒,阳气不足,脾胃失于温煦滋养,而见胃痛、食少等症。

can be seen.

5. Stagnation of qi leading to a local obstruction

Gastropathy with long-standing case, repeated attack, stagnation of qi and blood in the stomach; or emotional upset, stagnation of the liver-qi, qi-stagnancy and blood stasis, blood stasis stagnating in channels and vessels marked by fixed stomachache and gastric fullness.

6. Heat transformed from dampness, blockage of the middle energizer

Over-drinking, or being addicted to eating greasy food, blockage of the middle energizer, resulting in dampness and heat, damage of the stomach and intestine; or the hyperactive liver-qi attacking the stomach, incoordination between the spleen and the stomach, resulting in dampness and heat; or exogenous cold dampness, invasion of the spleen and stomach, retention of dampness in the interior, resulting in the dampness and heat, leading to dampness and heat blocking the middle energizer, thoracic fullness, bitter taste, stomachache and pantothenic acid.

5. 气滞不行,瘀血内阻

胃病日久,反复发作,经久不愈,气血瘀阻胃脘;或者情志不舒,肝郁气滞,气滞血瘀,瘀血阻滞留络,而见胃痛固定不移、脘腹胀满等症。

6. 湿蕴生热,阻滞中焦

嗜酒过度,或嗜食肥甘厚腻,阻滞中焦,酿湿生热,损伤胃肠;或因肝气犯胃,脾胃失和,蕴湿生热;或因外感寒湿,内侵脾胃,水湿内停,日久化生湿热,湿热中阻,而见痞满、口苦、胃痛、泛酸等症。

Part Two Characteristic Therapy

Chapter One The Treatment of Chronic Superficial Gastritis

Section One Internal therapy

1. Treatment based on differentiation of symptoms and signs

(1) Retention of food in the stomach

Symptoms and signs: There is a clear history of impairment by overeating and anorexia. There is nausea and vomiting when eating with the symptoms of abdominal distention, dirty air from the mouth, smelly and loose stool, bright red tongue, greasy fur, slippery powerful and rapid pulse.

Therapeutic methods: Improving digestion and removing food retention.

Recipe: Modified Baohe Pill. Ingredients: Shenqu, Laifuzi, Shanzha, Banxia, Chenpi and Fuling, etc. If there are epigastralgia, fullness and constipation, Shengdahuang, Muxiang and Zhishi are added.

中篇 特色疗法

一、慢性浅表性胃炎的治疗

（一）内治疗法

1. 辨证治疗

（1）食滞胃脘

【证候】 有明显伤食病史，不思饮食，食则恶心欲吐，甚者厌食，脘腹胀满，口出秽腐之气，大便腐臭，溏而不爽，舌质红暗、苔厚腻，脉滑数有力。

【治法】 消食化滞。

【方药】 保和丸加味。药用神曲、莱菔子、山楂、半夏、陈皮、茯苓等。若胃脘胀痛而便秘者，可加生大黄、木香、枳实等。

(2) Simultaneous disease of the pharynx and stomach

Symptoms and signs: Most of the patients have the history of chronic pharyngitis. The symptoms include sensation of a foreign body in the throat; difficulty in throwing up and swallowing; chest distress; fullness in the stomach; belching again and again; food subjectively reflux to pharyngeal portion; dysphoria and easy to anger; purplish red tongue, white thin lingual fur or greasy, thin taut pulse.

Therapeutic methods: Regulating qi and stomach, relieving sore-throat and eliminating stagnation.

Recipe: Modified Banxia Houpo Decoction. Ingredients: Banxia, Fuling, Houpo, Zisugeng and Shengjiang, etc. If there is throat discomfort, Muhudie and Jiegeng are added.

(3) Hepatic qi attacking the stomach

Symptoms and signs: Fullness and pain in the stomach, hypochondrium pain, exacerbation with nausea and vomiting, frequent belching, comfortable in breaking wind, easy to sigh, pale red tongue, white thin lingual fur, taut pulse.

Therapeutic methods: Soothing the liver and harmonizing the stomach, regulating qi to relieve depression.

Recipe: Modified Chaihu Shugan Powder. Ingredients: Chaihu, Baishaoyao, Gancao, Chuanxiong, Zhi-

（2）咽胃同病

【证候】 多有慢性咽炎病史，咽喉有异物感，吐之不出，咽之不下，胸闷不舒，胃脘胀满，嗳气频作，自觉有食物反流至咽部，时有心烦易怒，舌质紫红、苔薄白或腻，脉细弦。

【治法】 理气和胃，利咽散结。

【方药】 半夏厚朴汤加减。药用半夏、茯苓、厚朴、紫苏梗、生姜等。咽喉不利者，加木蝴蝶、桔梗等。

（3）肝气犯胃

【证候】 胃脘胀满疼痛，痛及两胁，逢情志不舒则加剧，兼见恶心呕吐，嗳气频繁，得矢气则舒，善太息，舌质淡暗、苔薄白，脉弦。

【治法】 疏肝和胃，理气解郁。

【方药】 柴胡疏肝散加减。药用柴胡、白芍药、甘草、川芎、制香附、

xiangfu, Chenpi and Yujin. If there is thirst and bitter taste in the mouth, Huanglian and Shanzhizi are added.

(4) Deficiency of the spleen and stomach

Symptoms and signs: Vague pain in the stomach, relief by warm and pressing, discomfort by turgor with exacerbation after meal, anorexia, hunger without appetite, cacochroia, mental fatigue and weakness, lassitude, loose stool, pale and fat tongue, white or greasy fur, slow and weakness pulse.

Therapeutic methods: Nourishing qi to invigorate the spleen, regulating and invigorating the stomach.

Recipe: Modified Yigong Powder. Ingredients: Dangshen (or Renshen), Baizhu, Fuling, Chenpi, Gancao, Dazao and Shengjiang. If there is dyspepsia Laifuzi and Maiya are added; if there is deficiency of both qi and blood, Goujizi is added; if there is bleeding, Sanqi and Baiji are added.

(5) Deficiency of gastric yin

Symptoms and signs: Vague pain in stomach, gastric upset, hunger without appetite, local feeling of burning usually exacerbation in the afternoon and fasting, dry mouth and lack of body fluid, belching and dry vomiting, constipation, red tongue, little fur, thin and rapid pulse.

Therapeutic methods: Nourishing gastric yin, promoting fluid production to clear away heat.

陈皮、郁金等。若口干而苦者,加黄连、山栀子等。

(4)脾胃虚弱

【证候】 胃脘隐隐作痛,喜温喜按,胀满不适,食后更甚,纳食减少,知饥不欲食,面色无华,神疲乏力,精神不振,大便溏薄,舌质淡胖、苔白或腻,脉缓无力。

【治法】 益气补脾,和中健胃。

【方药】 异功散加减。药用党参(或人参)、白术、茯苓、陈皮、甘草、大枣、生姜等。若挟有食滞者,加莱菔子、麦芽等以消食导滞;气血两虚者,加枸杞子以益气补血;兼出血者,加参三七、白及以化瘀止血。

(5)胃阴不足

【证候】 胃脘隐痛,嘈杂似饥,饥不欲食,局部有灼热感,多在午后、空腹时为重,口干少津,嗳气干呕,大便干结,舌质红、少苔,脉细数。

【治法】 滋阴养胃,生津清热。

Recipe: Modified Yiwei Decoction. Ingredients: Shashen, Maimendong, Shengdihuang, Yuzhu and Bingtang. If there is blood stasis and drastic epigastralgia, Wulingzhi and Shengpuhuang are added; if there is fullness in the stomach, Xiangyuan, Foshou, Daidaihua and Meiguihua are added.

(6) Asthenia of splenogastric yang

Symptoms and signs: Vague pain in stomach, lingering pain for long time, relief by warm and pressing, anorexia and gastric cavity painful abdominal mass, vomiting water, cool hands and feet, cold trunk and limbs, lassitude and mental fatigue, pale, loose stool or diarrhea with undigested food in the stool, white pale and tender tongue, white watering fur, sunken and thin pulse with weakness or sunken and retarded pulse.

Therapeutic methods: Warming the middle energizer and strengthening the spleen, warming the stomach to eliminate cold.

Recipe: Modified Huangqi Jianzhong Decoction and Lizhong Decoction. Ingredients: Dangshen, Baizhu, Paojiang, Sharen, Muxiang, Huangqi, Baishaoyao, Guizhi, Gancao, Ganjiang, Muxiang and Dazao. If there is pale complexion, Danggui is added; if there is obvious pain in the stomach, Chaopuhuang and Sanqifen are added.

(7) Blood stasis blocking the stomach

【方药】　益胃汤加减。药用沙参、麦门冬、生地黄、玉竹、冰糖等。若挟瘀血，胃痛较剧者，加五灵脂、生蒲黄以化瘀止痛；胃脘胀闷不适者，加入香橼、佛手、玳玳花、玫瑰花等理气而不伤阴之品。

（6）脾胃虚寒

【证候】　胃脘隐痛，痛势缠绵，持续不已，喜温喜按，纳少脘痞，泛吐清水，手足不温，形寒肢冷，倦怠神疲，面色苍白，大便溏薄，或下利清谷，舌质淡白而嫩、苔白或水滑，脉沉细无力，或沉迟。

【治法】　温中健脾，暖胃散寒。

【方药】　黄芪建中汤、理中汤加减。药用党参、白术、炮姜、砂仁、木香、黄芪、白芍药、桂枝、甘草、干姜、木香、大枣等。面色苍白者，加当归以养血活血；胃脘痛明显者，加炒蒲黄、三七粉以化瘀止痛。

（7）瘀血阻胃

Symptoms and signs: Pain as needling in stomach, exacerbation at night, pain fixed in one place and unpressable, hunger without appetite, difficult belching, dysphoria and sleeplessness, dark purplish tongue with ecchymosis and petechia, or blue veins visible on the tongue, sunken and unsmooth pulse.

Therapeutic methods: Regulating qi and activating blood, eliminating stasis to stop pain.

Recipe: Modified Shixiao Powder. Ingredients: Puhuang, Wulingzhi, Danggui, Chishaoyao, Yanhusuo and Danshen, etc. If there are symptoms of qi deficiency, anorexia and mental fatigue, Huangqi and Huangjing are added; if there are symptoms of blood stasis, qi stagnation and drastic pain, Wuyao and Xiangfu are added for regulating Qi and promoting blood flow.

(8) Damp-heat in the spleen and stomach

Symptoms and signs: Gastric cavity fullness or pain, belching and nausea, gastric upset and pantothenic acid, turbid qi from the mouth, bitter taste and dry of mouth, anorexia and physical fatigue, dizziness and insomnia, dry mouth without desire to drink, unsmooth defecation, brown and turbid urine, red tongue, yellowish and greasy fur, soft rapid or taut slippery pulse.

Therapeutic methods: Clearing away heat and eliminating dampness, regulating qi to harmonize the stomach.

【证候】 胃脘疼痛,痛如针刺,夜间为甚,痛处固定,拒按,饥而不欲食,嗳气不爽,心烦少寐,舌质紫暗,有瘀斑瘀点,或舌下青筋暴露,脉沉涩。

【治法】 理气活血,化瘀止痛。

【方药】 失笑散加味。药用蒲黄、五灵脂、当归、赤芍药、延胡索、丹参等。若兼有气虚,食少神疲者,加黄芪、黄精以益气;血瘀气滞,疼痛较剧者,加入乌药、香附等理气药物,气行则血行。

（8）脾胃湿热

【证候】 胃脘痞满或疼痛,嗳气恶心,嘈杂泛酸,口出浊气,口苦而干,纳少身困,头晕寐差,渴不思饮,大便不畅,小便黄浊,舌质红、苔黄腻,脉濡数或弦滑。

【治法】 清化湿热,理气和胃。

Recipe: Modified Banxia Xiexin Decoction. Ingredients: Huanglian, Huangqin, Jiaozhizi, Chenpi, Banxia, Fuling, Houpo, Huoxiang, Cangzhu and Gancao, etc. If there is obvious anorexia, Jineijin, Shenqu and Maiya are added to promotion digestion to eliminate stagnation.

2. Chinese patent medicines

(1) Baohe Pill

Ingredients: Shanzha, Liushenqu, Banxia, Fuling, Chenpi, Lianqiao, Laifuzi and Maiya.

Functions: Promoting digestion to eliminate stagnation.

Indications: Fullness in stomach resulting from dyspepsia, fetid eructation and anorexia, gastric upset, etc.

Direction: 6 - 9 g, per time, twice a day, 1/2 adult dosage for children of seven. Avoiding greasy and stinking food.

(2) Shanzha Jianpi Pill

Ingredients: Shanzha, Shanyao, Baibiandou, Qianshi, Yiyiren, Liushenqu, Maiya, Lianzirou and Fuling.

Functions: Invigorating the spleen to promote digestion, regulating qi and eliminating dampness.

Indications: Food retention due to spleen deficiency marked by fullness in the epigastric region, distending pain, etc.

【方药】 半夏泻心汤加减。药用黄连、黄芩、焦栀子、陈皮、半夏、茯苓、厚朴、藿香、苍术、甘草等。食欲不振明显者,加鸡内金、神曲、麦芽以消食导滞。

2. 中成药

（1）保和丸

【组成】 山楂、六神曲、半夏、茯苓、陈皮、连翘、莱菔子、麦芽。

【功用】 消食导滞。

【适应证】 食滞引起的脘腹胀满、嗳腐厌食、嘈杂不适等。

【用法】 每次 6～9 g,每日 2 次。7 岁以上儿童服成人 1/2 量,3～7 岁服成人 1/3 量。忌油腻腥黏等物。

（2）山楂健脾丸

【组成】 山楂、山药、白扁豆、芡实、薏苡仁、六神曲、麦芽、莲子肉、茯苓。

【功效】 健脾消食,理气化湿。

【适应证】 脾虚积滞内停引起的脘腹痞满、胀痛等。

Direction: 2 pills per time, twice a day.

(3) Binglang Sixiao Pill

Ingredients: Mangxiao, Qianniuzi, Binglang, Zhike, Sharen, Chenpi, Maiya, Shanzha, Muxiang, Houpo, Xiangfu, Dahuang, Qingpi and Huangqin.

Functions: Regulating qi, eliminating stagnation and alleviating water retention.

Indications: Fullness in the epigastric region, nausea and vomiting caused by indigestion and phlegmatic retention.

Direction: 6 g per time, twice a day.

(4) Kaixiong Shunqi Pill

Ingredients: Qianniuzi, Muxiang, Binglang, Chenpi, Houpo, Sanleng, Ezhu and Zhuyazao.

Functions: Regulating qi and removing food retention, eliminating stagnation to stop pain.

Indications: Hepatic and gastric qi stagnation, food stasis, gastric distending pain, etc.

Direction: 3 - 6 g per time, twice a day.

(5) Liangfu Pill

Ingredients: Gaoliangjiang and Xiangfu.

Functions: Warming the middle energizer to dispel cold, regulating qi to stop pain.

Indications: Gastric pain and abdominal distension resulted from cold obstruction causing qi stagnation.

【用法】 每次2丸,每日2次。

（3）槟榔四消丸

【组成】 芒硝、牵牛子、槟榔、枳壳、砂仁、陈皮、麦芽、山楂、木香、厚朴、香附、大黄、青皮、黄芩。

【功效】 理气化滞行水。

【适应证】 食积痰饮所致的脘腹闷胀、恶心呕吐等。

【用法】 每次6g,每日2次。

（4）开胸顺气丸

【组成】 牵牛子、木香、槟榔、陈皮、厚朴、三棱、莪术、猪牙皂。

【功效】 理气消积,化滞止痛。

【适应证】 肝胃气滞,饮食停滞,胃脘胀痛等。

【用法】 每次3～6g,每日2次。

（5）良附丸

【组成】 高良姜、香附。

【功效】 温中散寒,理气止痛。

【适应证】 寒凝气滞引起的胃脘疼痛、腹胀喜暖等。

Direction: 3 - 6 g per time, twice a day.

(6) Weiqitong Tablet

Ingredients: Wuyao, Yujin, Xiangfu, Gaoliangjiang and Qingpi.

Functions: Warming the stomach to dispel cold, regulating qi to stop pain.

Indications: Gastrofrigid pain, vomiting acid water, etc.

Direction: 5 tablets per time, twice a day.

(7) Shixiang Zhitong Pill

Ingredients: Dingxiang, Ruxiang, Moyao, Xiaohui-xiang, Bingpian, Chenxiang, Xiangfu, Tanxiang, Jiang-xiang, Guanghuoxiang and Shexiang (artificial).

Functions: Promoting qi to activate blood, eliminating cold to stop pain.

Indications: Gastric and abdominal distending pain resulted from qi stagnation and gastric cold.

Direction: 6 - 9 g per time, twice a day.

(8) Shugan Hewei Pill

Ingredients: Baizhu, Chenpi, Xiangfu, Foshou, Muxiang, Wuyao, Chaihu, Yujin, Guanghuoxiang, Baishaoyao, Gancao, Binglang and Laifuzi.

Functions: Relaxing the liver and regulating the stomach, promoting qi to stop pain.

Indications: Qi stagnating in liver and stomach,

【用法】 每次3～6 g,每日2次。

(6) 胃气痛片

【组成】 乌药、郁金、香附、高良姜、青皮。

【功效】 温胃散寒,理气止痛。

【适应证】 胃寒疼痛,呕吐酸水等。

【用法】 每次5片,每日2次。

(7) 十香止痛丸

【组成】 丁香、乳香、没药、小茴香、冰片、沉香、香附、檀香、降香、广藿香、麝香(人工)。

【功效】 行气活血,散寒止痛。

【适应证】 气滞胃寒所致的脘腹胀痛等。

【用法】 每次6～9 g,每日2次。

(8) 舒肝和胃丸

【组成】 白术、陈皮、香附、佛手、木香、乌药、柴胡、郁金、广藿香、白芍药、甘草、槟榔、莱菔子等。

【功效】 舒肝和胃,行气止痛。

【适应证】 肝胃气滞不舒,脘胀

gastric disending and belching.

Direction: One pill, twice a day.

(9) Chenxiang Shuqi Pill

Ingredients: Chenxiang, Houpo, Zhike and Caodoukou.

Functions: Regulating qi to stop pain, strengthening stomach to eliminate stagnation.

Indications: Qi stagnation in the liver and stomach, dyspepsia in the interior.

Direction: 6 g per time, twice a day.

(10) Yanhu Zhitong Tablet

Ingredients: Yanhusuo and Baizhi.

Functions: Regulating qi and activating blood to stop pain.

Indications: Epigastralgia resulted from qi stagnation and blood stasis.

Direction: 4 - 6 tablets per time, twice a day.

(11) Zhishi Xiaopi Pill

Ingredients: Dangshen, Baizhu, Gancao, Ganjiang, Zhishi, Huanglian, Houpo, Maiya and Banxia.

Functions: Invigorating spleen to eliminate dampness, eliminating abdominal mass to relieve distension.

Indications: Internal blocking with dampness food resulted from spleen deficiency, thoracic fullness and anorexia, abdominal distention and greasy fur,etc.

嗳气等。

【用法】 每次1丸,每日2次。

(9) 沉香舒气丸

【组成】 沉香、厚朴、枳壳、草豆蔻等。

【功效】 理气止痛,健胃消积。

【适应证】 肝胃气滞、积滞内停之证。

【用法】 每次6g,每日2次。

(10) 延胡止痛片

【组成】 延胡索、白芷。

【功效】 理气活血止痛。

【适应证】 气滞血瘀引起的胃痛。

【用法】 每次4～6片,每日2次。

(11) 枳实消痞丸

【组成】 党参、白术、甘草、干姜、枳实、黄连、厚朴、麦芽、半夏。

【功效】 健脾除湿,化积消痞。

【适应证】 脾虚所致的湿食内阻,痞满恶食、腹胀、苔腻等。

Direction: 6 - 9 g per time, twice a day.

(12) Xiangsha Yangwei Pill

Ingredients: Baizhu, Houpo, Fuling, Banxia, Xiangfu, Sharen, Zhishi, Huoxiang, Baidoukou, Chenpi and Gancao.

Functions: Invigorating the spleen to nourish qi.

Indications: Qi deficiency in the spleen and stomach, vague pain in stomach, relieving after meal with fatigue, loose stool or diarrhea, etc.

Direction: 6 g per time, twice a day.

3. Simple and proved formulae

(1) Ziwei Decoction

Ingredients: Wumeirou 6 g, Chaobaishaoyao 10 g, Beishashen 10 g, Maimendong 10 g, Shihu 10 g, Danshen 10 g, Shengmaiya 10 g, Zhijineijin 5 g, Meiguihua 5 g, Zhigancao 3 g.

Functions: Nourishing yin and regulating the stomach.

Indications: Gastric yin deficiency in chronic superficial gastritis.

Direction: Simmer in water, one dose a day, twice a day.

(2) Baihua Gongying Decoction

Ingredients: Baihuasheshecao 30 g and Pugongying 30 g.

Functions: Clearing away heat to remove toxin.

【用法】 每次6～9 g,每日2次。

(12)香砂养胃丸

【组成】 白术、厚朴、茯苓、半夏、香附、砂仁、枳实、藿香、白豆蔻、陈皮、甘草。

【功效】 健脾益气。

【适应证】 脾胃气虚,胃脘隐痛不适,食后稍缓,伴有疲倦乏力,大便不实或溏薄等。

【用法】 每次6 g,每日2次。

3. 单方验方

(1)滋胃饮

【组成】 乌梅肉6 g,炒白芍药、北沙参、麦门冬、石斛、丹参、生麦芽各10 g,炙鸡内金、玫瑰花各5 g,炙甘草3 g。

【功用】 养阴和胃。

【适应证】 慢性浅表性胃炎胃阴不足者。

【用法】 水煎,每日1剂,分2次温服。

(2)白花公英饮

【组成】 白花蛇舌草30 g,蒲公英30 g。

【功用】 清热解毒。

Indications: Pathogenic heat a bit aggressive in chronic superficial gastritis.

Direction: To be infused into boiled water and drunk frequently.

(3) Yizhong Huoxue Decoction

Ingredients: Huangqi 30 g, Rougui 8 g, Wuzhuyu 10 g, Ruxiang 8 g, Moyao 8 g, Shengpuhuang 12 g, Sanleng 10 g, Ezhu 10 g, Chuanxiong 12 g, Wuyao 12 g and Danshen 15 g.

Functions: Nourishing qi and strengthening the spleen, activating blood to stop pain.

Indications: Middle energizer deficiency and blood stasis in chronic superficial gastritis.

Direction: Simmer in water, one dose a day, twice a day.

(4) Huoxue Huayu Decoction

Ingredients: Huangqi 10 g, Danggui 10 g, Chuanxiong 10 g, Zhike 10 g, Gaoliangjiang 6 g, Ruxiang 8 g, Moyao 8 g, Zhigancao 3 g.

Functions: Activating blood to remove blood stasis to stop pain.

Indications: Incurable long-standing case in chronic superficial gastritis with clearly blood stasis.

Direction: Simmer in water, one dose a day, twice a day.

【适应证】 慢性浅表性胃炎热邪偏盛者。

【用法】 开水冲泡频饮。

(3) 益中活血汤

【组成】 黄芪 30 g,肉桂 8 g,吴茱萸 10 g,乳香、没药各 8 g,生蒲黄 12 g,三棱、莪术各 10 g,川芎、乌药各 12 g,丹参 15 g。

【功用】 益气健脾,活血止痛。

【适应证】 慢性浅表性胃炎中虚血瘀者。

【用法】 水煎,每日 1 剂,分 2 次温服。

(4) 活血化瘀汤

【组成】 黄芪、当归、川芎、枳壳各 10 g,高良姜 6 g,乳香、没药各 8 g,炙甘草 3 g。

【功用】 活血化瘀止痛。

【适应证】 慢性浅表性胃炎病久不愈,血瘀较明显者。

【用法】 水煎,每日 1 剂,分 2 次温服。

（5）Wenwei Zhitong Decoction

Ingredients：Guizhi 5 g, Baishaoyao 9 g, Wuzhuyu 6 g, Dingxiang 3 g, Fuling 6 g, Sharen 5 g, Paojiang 5 g, Danggui 9 g, Yanhusuo 9 g, Baizhu 12 g, Dazao 3 pieces.

Functions：Warming the stomach to dissipate cold, regulating qi to relieve pain.

Indications：Evident stomachache of chronic superficial gastritis in the pattern of cold congealing and qi stagnation.

Direction：Decoct one packet of the herbs in water. Drink the decoction twice at a warm temperature every day.

（6）Zhang Jingren Zhi Manxing Weiyan Decoction

Ingredients：Chaihu, Chaobaishaoyao, Zhigancao, Shengbaizhu, Zisugeng, Pingdimu, Xuchangqing, Lianqiao, Bayuezha, Zhixiangfu.

Functions：Soothing the liver, regulating qi, clearing away heat and harmonizing the stomach.

Indications：Chronic superficial gastritis in the pattern of qi stagnation and heat depression.

Direction：Decoct one packet of the herbs in water. Drink the decoction twice at a warm temperature every day.

（7）Wubeizi Decoction

Ingredients：Wubeizi 1 piece, Xingren 7 pieces,

（5）温胃止痛汤

【组成】 桂枝 5 g,白芍药 9 g,吴茱萸 6 g,丁香 3 g,茯苓 6 g,砂仁 5 g,炮姜 5 g,当归 9 g,延胡索 9 g,白术 12 g,大枣3 枚。

【功用】 温胃散寒,理气止痛。

【适应证】 主治慢性浅表性胃炎寒凝气滞,胃痛较重者。

【用法】 水煎,每日 1 剂,分 2 次温服。

（6）张镜人治慢性胃炎方

【组成】 柴胡、炒白芍药、炙甘草、生白术、紫苏梗、平地木、徐长卿、连翘、八月札、制香附。

【功用】 疏肝理气,清热和胃。

【适应证】 慢性浅表性胃炎气滞郁热者。

【用法】 水煎,每日 1 剂,分 2 次温服。

（7）五倍子饮

【组成】 五倍子 1 个,杏仁 7

Dazao 7 pieces.

Functions: Astringing, harmonizing the stomach and checking acid.

Indications: Evident acid regurgitation of chronic superficial gastritis.

Direction: Decoct the herbs in water and drink the decoction for once.

(8) Bingpian Hujiao Powder

Ingredients: Bingpian 2.5 g, Hujiao 7 pieces.

Functions: Warming the stomach, dissipating cold and stopping pain.

Indications: Chronic superficial gastritis in the pattern of stomach cold.

Direction: Grind the herbs into fine powder and dissolve it in water for oral administration.

(9) Zhitong Powder

Ingredients: Yanhusuo 25 g, Wulingzhi 25 g, Caoguo 25 g, Moyao 25 g.

Functions: Removing stasis, regulating qi and stopping pain.

Indications: Stabbing gastric pain resulting from chronic superficial gastritis in the pattern of qi stagnation and blood stasis.

Direction: Grind the herbs into fine powder. Orally administrate the powder with warm Chinese liquor, as a

个,大枣 7 枚。

【功用】　收敛和胃止酸。

【适应证】　慢性浅表性胃炎胃酸较多者。

【用法】　水煎后,1 次饮用。

(8) 冰片胡椒散

【组成】　冰片 2.5 g,胡椒 7 粒。

【功用】　温中散寒止痛。

【适应证】　慢性浅表性胃炎属胃寒者。

【用法】　共研细末,白开水冲服。

(9) 止痛散

【组成】　延胡索、五灵脂、草果、没药各 25 g。

【功用】　化瘀理气止痛。

【适应证】　慢性浅表性胃炎气滞血瘀所致的胃脘疼痛,痛如针刺。

【用法】　研为细末,每次 15 g,每日 2 次,以白酒(温)为引,可加少

guide conductor, 15 g per time and twice a day. A little bit warm water can be added in the alcohol.

(10) Gancao Walengzi Powder

Ingredients: Same ratio of Walengzi and Gancao.

Functions: Harmonize the stomach and check acid.

Indications: Evident acid regurgitation of chronic superficial gastritis.

Direction: Grind herbs into fine powder. Orally administrate the powder 5 – 15 g per time and twice a day.

(11) Lianyu Powder

Ingredients: Wuzhuyu 20 g, Huanglian 6 g, Haipiaoxiao 15 g, Muli 15 g, Cangzhu 10 g.

Functions: Warming the stomach, drying dampness, clearing away heat and checking acid.

Indications: Chronic superficial gastritis in the pattern of cold-heat complex.

Direction: Grind the herbs into fine powder. Orally administrate the powder 12 g per time and three times a day.

Section Two　External treatment

1. Dressing therapies

(1) Fufang Wuzhuyu Paste

Wuzhuyu 50 g, Ganjiang 50 g, Dingxiang 50 g, Xiaohuixiang 75 g, Rougui 30 g, Shengliuhuang 30 g, Shanzhizi 20 g, Hujiao 5 g, Biba 25 g. Grind the herbs into powder and

量温开水。

（10）甘草瓦楞子散

【组成】　瓦楞子、甘草各等份。

【功用】　和胃止酸。

【适应证】　慢性浅表性胃炎胃酸分泌较多者。

【用法】　上两味共研为细末，每次服 5～15 g，每日 2 次，口服。

（11）连萸散

【组成】　吴茱萸 20 g，黄连 6 g，海螵蛸 15 g，牡蛎 15 g，苍术 10 g。

【功用】　温中燥湿，清热制酸。

【适应证】　慢性浅表性胃炎属寒热错杂者。

【用法】　上药研为细末，每次 12 g，每日 3 次，口服。

（二）外治疗法

1. 敷贴法

（1）复方吴茱萸糊

吴茱萸、干姜、丁香各 50 g，小茴香 75 g，肉桂、生硫黄各 30 g，山栀子 20 g，胡椒 5 g，荜茇 25 g，共研粉末，

restore the powder in an air-tight container for future use. Mix 25 g herbal powder with the same amount paste. Apply the paste on Shenque (CV 8) and fix it with adhesive plaster 3 - 6 hours per time and once or twice a day.

(2) Weitong Paste

Chuanjiao 150 g, Paojiang 100 g, Shengfuzi 100 g, Tanxiang 100 g, Cangzhu 200 g. Grind the herbs into fine powder and store the powder in a container for future use. Stir ginger juice with 30 g herbal powder until paste is formed. Apply the paste on Zhongwan (CV 12), Zusanli (ST 36), Shenque (CV 8), Pishu (BL 20) and Weishu (BL 21) once a day.

(3) Jianpi Ointment

Baizhu 120 g, Fuling 60 g, Baishaoyao 60 g, Shenqu 60 g, Maiya 60 g, Xiangfu 60 g, Danggui 60 g, Zhike 60 g, Banxia 60 g, Chenpi 20 g, Huanglian 21 g, Wuzhuyu 21 g, Shanzha 21 g, Baikouren 21 g, Yizhiren 21 g, Huangqi 21 g, Shanyao 21 g, Dangshen 15 g, Guangmuxiang 15 g, Gancao 21 g. Crush the herbs and fry them in a boiling sesame oil until they become burnt brown. After filtering the sediment, concentrate the decoction to thick gelatin, on which drops of water can form a pearl. Add Qiandan (main ingredient of which is Pb_3O_4) and stir the preparation evenly until ointment is formed. Apply it on Zhongwan (CV 12), Zusanli (ST 36), Shenque (CV 8), Pishu (BL 20) and Weishu (BL

密贮备用。治疗时取药末 25 g,加入等量面粉调成糊状,贴神阙穴,外用胶布固定,每次敷贴 3～6 小时,每日 1～2 次。

(2)胃痛糊

川椒 150 g,炮姜 100 g,生附子 100 g,檀香 100 g,苍术 200 g,共研细末,贮存备用。治疗时取药末 30 g,用生姜汁调成糊状,敷于中脘、足三里、神阙、脾俞、胃俞等。每日 1 次。

(3)健脾膏

白术 120 g,茯苓、白芍药、神曲、麦芽、香附、当归、枳壳、半夏各 60 g,陈皮 20 g,黄连、吴茱萸、山楂、白蔻仁、益智仁、黄芪、山药各 21 g,党参、广木香各 15 g,甘草 21 g,上药研碎,先将麻油加热至沸,再将上药放入炸枯,过滤去渣,再熬炼成稠膏状,至滴水成珠不散为度,再加入铅丹搅匀成膏,贴于中脘、足三里、神阙、脾俞、胃俞等穴位上,3 天更换 1 次。

21). Change it once every three days.

(4) Nuanwei Gao (Plaster)

Shengjiang 500 g, Niupijiao 15 g, Ruxiangmo 15 g, Moyao 15 g. Crush the ginger juice and decoct it with other herbs in the water until ointment is formed. Use ointment to make three large pieces of herbal plaster. Apply one piece of plaster, after being heated, on the stomachache position. It is beneficial to chronic gastritis with the presence of evident stomach discomfort, cold pain, and vomiting clear drool.

(5) Weitong Powder

Same ratio of Zhangnao, Xuejie, Ruxiang, Moyao, Biba, Wuzhuyu, Xixin, Muxiang, Dingxiang, Chaihu. Bake the herbs and grind them into powder. Stir tea or vinegar with the herbal powder until ointment is formed. Apply the ointment on Shangwan (CV 13), Zhongwan (CV 12), Xiawan (CV 10), Pishu (BL 20), Weishu (BL 21) and Liangmen (ST 21) for 8 hours every day. One week consists of one course. The formula is beneficial to chronic gastritis with the presence of upper abdominal pain, uncomfortable full sensation, belching, and reduced intake of food.

(6) Supplemented Xiexin Paste

Huanglian 7 g, Ganjiang 8 g, Banxia 6 g, Gancao 6 g, Huangqin 10 g, Dazao 10 g, Dangshen 20 g, furazolidone 2 g

(4) 暖胃膏

生姜 500 g,捣取汁,入牛皮胶、乳香末、没药各 15 g,水煎,胶化离火,将药作三张大膏药。取一张贴胃脘痛处,并加热熨之。适用于慢性胃炎以胃脘不适、冷痛、呕吐清涎为主症者。

(5) 胃痛散

樟脑、血竭、乳香、没药、荜茇、吴茱萸、细辛、木香、丁香、柴胡各等份,烘干共研细末,以茶水或醋搅拌成膏,敷贴上、中、下三脘穴,脾俞、胃俞穴,梁门穴。每日 1 次,每次贴 8 小时后取下,1 周为 1 个疗程。本方适用于慢性胃炎,症见上腹疼痛、饱胀不适、嗳气纳少者。

(6) 加味泻心糊

黄连 7 g,干姜 8 g,半夏 6 g,甘草 6 g,黄芩 10 g,大枣 10 g,党参 20 g,

and proglumide 4 g. Grind the herbs into powder and store it in a bottle for future use. Stir 75% alcohol (or Chinese liquor) with duly amount herbal powder until paste is formed. Apply it, once every day, on the umbilicus and fix it with Shang Shi Zhi Tong Gao (plaster) or adhesive plaster. Ten days consist of a course. Five-day interval is between two courses. It can also vary the course from 1 to 4 according to the stage of the disease.

2. Vesiculation therapies

Select fresh Maolang. Cut the leave and stem but keep the root hair. Crush it after cleaning in water. Add 30% brown sugar and break them completely. Put them in the inner indentation of the rubber lid of penicillin ampules. Put the ampules on Weishu (BL 21) and Shenshu (BL 23) for about 15 minutes. Take it off when the patient has baking feverish sensation on local skin. If the vesicles are formed on the skin, it will be absorbed naturally without the damage by the needle. The method is mainly for the evident stomachache of chronic superficial gastritis.

3. Herbal plaster therapies

(1) Pingweisan Jiawei Wenwei Plaster

Cangzhu, Houpo, Chenpi, Gancao, Baizhu, Shenqu, Maiya, Huanglian, Wuzhuyu, Xiangfu, Zhike, Zhishi, Gaoliangjiang, Rougui, Baishaoyao, Danggui, (same ratio). Stir-fry the herbs in sesame oil and

痢特灵 2 g,丙谷胺 4 g,共研末贮瓶备用。用时取适量药末与 75% 的酒精(白酒亦可)调成糊状,敷于脐中,用伤湿止痛膏或胶布固定。每日换药 1 次,10 日为 1 个疗程,每疗程间隔 5 天,亦可根据病情确定疗程,一般 1～4 个疗程不等。

2. 发泡法

取鲜毛茛,除去叶、茎,留下根须,清水洗净,然后切碎,加入约 30% 红糖,捣烂,装入青霉素瓶橡皮盖凹槽内,敷贴胃俞、肾俞穴,置 15 分钟左右。局部有烘热感时揭去,如发生水泡,不必刺破,让其自行吸收。本方主治慢性浅表性胃炎以胃痛为主症者。

3. 膏药法

(1) 平胃散加味温胃膏

苍术、厚朴、陈皮、甘草、白术、神曲、麦芽、黄连、吴茱萸、香附、枳壳、枳实、高良姜、肉桂、白芍药、当归各等份,麻油熬,铅丹收,分摊膏药。贴

concentrate with Qiandan until it thick ointment is formed. Spread the ointment on the plaster and adhere one or two pieces on Shangwan (CV 13), Zhongwan (CV 12) and Xiawan (CV 10), or umbilicus once every week. The method is mainly used for gastritis in the pattern of stomach cold with the presence of discomfort of fullness and distention, or dull pain in the upper abdomen, aggravation after catching cold, no desire to eat, nausea and vomiting, belching, or usually accompanied with sloppy diarrhea, white fur and moderate pulse.

(2) Qingwei Plaster

Shengjiang100 g, Chenpi 100 g, Shichangpu 30 g, Congbai 60 g, Jiubai 60 g, Xiebai 60 g, Huoxiang 60 g, Baimaogen 120 g, Sangye 120 g, Pipaye 120 g, Zhuye 120 g, Huaizhi 240 g, Liuzhi 240 g, Sangzhi 240 g, Juhua 240 g, Wumei 3 pieces. Stir-fry the herbs in sesame oil and concentrate with qian dan. Then add Shengshigao 240 g, Hanshuishi 120 g, Qingdai 3 g, Mulifen 100 g, Mangxiao 100 g, Niupijiao 120 g and steam all the herbs with alcohol. Spread the medicinal on the plaster and adhere one or two pieces on Shangwan (CV 13), Zhongwan (CV 12) and Xiawan (CV 10) or umbilicus every seven days. The method is mainly used for gastritis in the pattern of stomach heat with the presence of paroxysmal burning pain in the upper abdomen, acid regurgitation, clamoring stomach, nausea and vomiting, or gastric bleeding,

上、中、下三脘穴或脐,每次贴
1～2张,7日更换1张。本方主治胃
寒型胃炎,症见上腹部胀满不适或隐
痛,遇寒较甚,不思饮食,恶心呕吐、
嗳气,或常伴大便溏泄,苔白、脉缓
者。

(2)清胃膏

生姜 100 g,陈皮 100 g,石菖蒲
30 g,葱白 60 g,韭白 60 g,薤白 60 g,
藿香 60 g,白茅根 120 g,桑叶 120 g,
枇杷叶 120 g,竹叶 120 g,槐枝 240 g,
柳枝 240 g,桑枝 240 g,菊花 240 g,乌
梅 3 个,麻油熬,铅丹收,再入生石膏
240 g,寒水石 120 g,青黛 3 g,牡蛎
粉、芒硝各 100 g,牛皮胶 120 g,酒蒸
化下,分摊膏药。贴上、中、下三脘穴
或脐,每次贴 1～2张,7日更换 1张。
本方主治胃热型胃炎,症见上腹部灼
热疼痛阵作、泛酸嘈杂、恶心呕吐,或
胃出血、心烦易怒、口干口苦,或大便
溏泄热臭,或大便秘结,或兼身热恶

vexation and irascibility, dry mouth and bitter taste in the mouth, or hot stinking sloppy diarrhea, or constipation, or generalized fever, aversion to cold, red tongue, and yellow or thick fur.

4. Hot compressing therapies

(1) Laifuzi Shengjiang Yun

Stir-fry duly amount Laifuzi with ginger until hot. Wrap the hot herbs with cloth and put the warm cloth on the upper abdomen. The method is for gastritis in the pattern of food accumulation with the presence of bloated distention in stomach duct, aggravation after intake of food, nausea and vomiting, and slimy fur.

(2) Lianxu Congtou Shengjiang Yun

green onion with root hair 30 g, fresh ginger 15 g. Crush and stir-fry two herbs until hot. Hot pack on the stomach region. Change the pack when it is cold. Do it twice a day. Each time is about 30 minutes or until the alleviation of pain.

5. Abdominal covering therapies

Biba 15 g, Ganjiang 15 g, Gansong 10 g, Shannai 10 g, Rougui 10 g, Wuzhuyu 10 g, Baizhi 10 g, Dahuixiang 6 g, Aiye 30 g. Grind the herbs into fine powder. Fold the soft cloth 40 cm×40 cm to a packet of the size of 20 cm×20 cm and put a layer of thin cotton inside. Scatter the powder evenly inside the packet and seal the packet with thread in

寒,舌红、苔黄或厚者。

4. 热熨法

（1）莱菔子生姜熨

莱菔子适量加生姜炒热布包温熨上腹部。适用于积滞型胃炎,症见胃脘饱胀、食入更甚、恶心呕吐、苔腻者。

（2）连须葱头生姜熨

连须葱头 30 g,生姜 15 g,两味共捣烂炒烫,热熨胃脘部,药袋冷即更换。每日 2 次,每次 30 分钟,或以疼痛缓解为度。

5. 兜肚法

荜茇 15 g,干姜 15 g,甘松 10 g,山柰 10 g,肉桂 10 g,吴茱萸 10 g,白芷 10 g,大茴香 6 g,艾叶 30 g,共研细末,用柔软的棉布 40 cm 折成 20 cm 见方的布兜,内铺一薄层棉花,将药均匀撒上,用线密密缝好,以防止药

case of the pile up and leakage of the powder. Apply the internal side of the packet closely to the skin on the stomach duct area. Change the powder once every 1 – 2 month. The method is for deficiency cold stomachache.

Section Three   Acumoxa therapies

1. Body acupuncture

Choose the points mainly on the conception vessel and foot yangming channels. Use the drainage manipulation for repletion patterns and the supplementation manipulation for deficiency patterns. Zhongwan (CV 12), Pishu (BL 20), Zusanli (ST 36) and Neiguan (PC 6) are the major points. Add Xiawan (CV10), Jianli (CV 11), and Neiting (ST 44) for food accumulation damaging the stomach. Add Neiting (ST 44), and Yanglingquan (GB 34) for stomach heat. Add Qimen (LR 14), Taichong (LR 3), and Yanglingquan (GB 34) for liver qi assailing the stomach. Add Pishu (BL 20), Weishu (BL 21), Sanyinjiao (SP 6) and Gongsun (SP 4) for the deficiency and weakness of spleen and stomach.

2. Moxibustion

Zhongwan (CV 12), Zusanli (ST 36), Pishu (BL 20) and Weishu (BL 21) are the major points. Add Shenque (CV 8), and Gongsun (SP 4) for abdominal cold pain. Add Shangwan (CV 13) and Guanyuan (CV 4) for

末堆积或漏出,将兜放在胃脘部,药兜内层紧贴皮肤,1～2个月换药1次。适用于脾胃虚寒型胃痛。

(三)针灸疗法

1. 体针

取任脉、足阳明经穴为主。针刺实证用泻法,虚证用补法,以中脘、脾俞、足三里、内关等为主穴。食积伤胃者加下脘、建里、内庭;胃热者加内庭、阳陵泉;肝气犯胃者加期门、太冲、阳陵泉;脾胃虚弱者加脾俞、胃俞、三阴交、公孙。

2. 灸法

主穴为中脘、足三里、脾俞、胃俞。腹中冷痛,加灸神阙、公孙;恶心呕吐,加灸上脘、关元;大便泄泻,加灸天枢、大肠俞。每日灸1次,每次

nausea and vomiting. Add Tianshu (ST 25), and Dachang-shu (BL 25) for diarrhea. Apply the moxibustion 10 – 30 minutes per time and once every day.

3. Ear acupuncture

Stomach, spleen, sympathetic nerve, and Shenmen are the major points. Add subcortex, and diaphragm for nausea and vomiting. Add liver for liver and stomach disharmony. Add pancreas and gallbladder for indigestion. Select 2 – 3 points in one treatment. Use strong stimulation for severe pain and mild stimulation for alleviated pain. Manipulate the needle intermittently. Remain the needle for 20 – 30 minutes. Change the points once every day or every other day.

4. Acupressure on ear points by Wangbuliuxingzi

Select points of Shenmen, sympathetic nerve, subcortex, spleen, cardiac orifice, diaphragm, stomach and intestines, liver, and gallbladder. Cut the plaster into the size of 2.5 cm × 0.8 cm, and 0.8 cm × 0.8 cm. Adhere 3 pieces of Wangbuliuxing with even distance on the longer plaster and 1 piece on the shorter one. Put longer plasters on cardiac orifice, diaphragm, stomach and intestines, shorter and longer plasters on liver and gallbladder, and shorter plaster on the other points. Press the points 6 – 8 times every other day from both sides of the ear. Each pressure lasts for 2 – 3 minutes. Or press the points when-

10～30 分钟。

3. 耳针

主穴为胃、脾、交感、神门。恶心呕吐加皮质下、膈;肝胃不和加肝;消化不良加胰、胆。每次选 2～3 穴,疼痛剧烈时用强刺激,疼痛缓解时用轻刺激,间歇行针,留针 20～30 分钟,隔日或每日 1 次。

4. 王不留行子耳压法

取穴为神门、交感、皮质下、脾、贲门、食道、胃肠、肝、胆等。先将胶布剪成 2.5 cm×0.8 cm 及 0.8 cm×0.8 cm 两种,前者黏 3 粒王不留行子,等距离;后者黏 1 粒。贲门、食道和胃、肠均用长条,肝、胆贴长、短条,余均贴短条。耳背对压,隔日 1 次,每日按压 6～8 次,每 2～3 分钟或痛时即按。

ever pain occurs.

5. Point injection

Select Zhongwan (CV 12), Liangmen (ST 21), Neiguan (PC 6), Zusanli (ST 36) and Yanglingquan (GB 34). Inject 0.5 - 1 ml Xuchangqing injection fluid, Danggui injection fluid, or vitamin B_1 injection fluid in 2 - 3 points once every other day. Ten days are one course.

6. Scalp acupuncture

Put the needle into bilateral stomach areas. Twist the needle in a high frequency and low amplitude for 2 - 3 minutes. Remain the needles for 5 - 10 minutes. Repeat the manipulation three times and withdraw the needles.

7. Plum blossom needle therapies

Tap the needle, in a moderate stimulating amplitude, the points of bilateral sides of $T_6 - T_{12}$, upper abdominal region, foot yangming channels, bladder channels, Zhongwan (CV 12), and Zusanli (ST 36) until the skin becomes reddening. Do the method once every day or every other day. Ten times consist of one course.

8. Needle embedding therapies

Alternatively select the pair points of Liangmen (ST 21) to Neiguan (PC 6), Shangwan (CV 13) to Zhongwan (CV 12), and Pishu (BL 20) to Weishu (BL 21). There are two ways. a. Catgut Embedding by

5. 穴位注射

取中脘、梁门、内关、足三里、阳陵泉,可酌情选用徐长卿注射液、当归注射液、维生素 B_1 注射液,每次选2~3穴,每穴注入药液 0.5~1 ml,隔日 1 次,10 日为 1 个疗程。

6. 头针

选双侧胃区,按头针操作常规,将针刺入后,用小幅度快频率捻转2~3分钟,留针 5~10 分钟,作第二次运针,方法如前,反复操作 3 次后,即可出针。

7. 梅花针

取胸椎 6~12 两侧、上腹、足阳明、膀胱及中脘、足三里等穴,中等量刺激至皮肤潮红,每日或隔日 1 次,10 次为 1 个疗程。

8. 埋线

取穴为梁门透内关、上脘透中脘、脾俞透胃俞,轮流使用。方法有两种:一种是穿刺针埋线:常规消毒局部皮肤,镊取一段 1~2 cm 长已消

Puncture Needle: Regularly sterilize the local skin. Pick up 1 - 2 cm sterilized catgut and put it at the tip of the lumbar puncture needle which is connected with stylet in the back. Stretch or pinch up the skin by left thumb and index finger. The right hand holds the syringe and penetrates the skin to the required depth. After patients have gained the needling sensation, push the stylet further and simultaneously withdraw the syringe. Embed the catgut in the subcutaneous tissue or muscles beneath the point. Cover the puncture holes with disinfectant gauze. b. Catgut Embedding by Triangular Suture Needle: Mark the location, 1 - 1. 5 cm bilateral to the points to insert the needle, by gentian violet. After sterilization, conduct the intradermal anesthesia by 0. 5% - 1% procaine in the marked spot. Use the needle holder to clenche the suture needle with catgut. Insert the needle from one side anesthetic spot, penetrating the subcutaneous tissue and muscles under the point, and emerge from the other side. Pinch up the skin between the two points. Cut the suture of both sides which are closed to the skin. Relax the skin and massage the local area gently until the catgut is fully buried in the intradermal tissue. Cover the points by gauze. It can select 1 - 3 location in one treatment. Do one treatment every 20 - 30 days.

毒的羊肠线,放置在腰椎穿刺针管的前端,后接针芯,左手拇、食指绷紧或捏起进针部位皮肤,右手拿针,刺入皮肤至所需要的深度;出现针感后,边推针芯,边退针管,将羊肠线埋植在穴位的皮下组织或肌层内,针孔处敷盖消毒纱布。另一种是三角缝针埋线:在距离穴位两侧 1～1.5 cm处,用龙胆紫作进出针点的标记。皮肤消毒后,在标记处用 0.5%～1% 的普鲁卡因作皮内麻醉。用持针器夹住带羊肠线的皮肤缝合针,从一侧局麻点刺入,穿过穴位下方的皮下组织或肌层,从对侧局麻点穿出。捏起两针孔之间的皮肤,紧贴皮肤剪断两端线头,放松皮肤,轻轻揉按局部,使肠线完全埋入皮下组织里。敷盖纱布。每次可用 1～3 个部位,一般 20～30 天埋线 1 次。

Section Four   Chinese massage (Tuina) therapies

1. Finger-press method

The patient lies on the bed and naturally crosses his hands on his forehead or below his chin. The doctor stands at one side of the patient and press Zhiyang (GV 9) (depression below the tubercle process of T_7) and Jizhong (GV 6) by the belly of both thumbs. Press and knead the two points in a circle for 1 – 5 minutes. Release the pressure until the patient can't tolerate. At the same time let the patient make even and deep abdominal breath. The method is for the cold stomachache.

2. Pressing and kneading on abdomen

Press the stomach area gently with hand. Trembling manipulation is also used if the patient has upper abdominal distention. Then press and knead clockwise around the umbilicus, from up to down, from right to left. Gently and rhythmically release the pressure while pressing and kneading. Do the method 20 minutes per time and once or twice a day.

3. Patting and sinew pinching method

Knead the tender spots gently on patient's back, which is just opposite to the tender spots of the stomach, for 3 – 5 minutes. Then knead gently below the xiphous process by four fingers. And finally pat the tender spots

（四）推拿按摩疗法

1. 指压法

患者俯卧，双手自然交错于头前或额下，术者位于患者一侧，用双手拇指指腹分别按压于至阳（第七胸椎棘突下凹陷中）与脊中穴，并在此两穴上作圆圈状按揉 1～5 分钟，用力以患者能忍受为度，同时令患者作均匀深长的腹式呼吸。本法适用于寒性胃痛。

2. 按摩腹部

用手轻轻按摩胃区，如上腹胀可用震颤手法，然后围绕脐部顺时针作环形揉按，从下而上，从右而左，并在揉按过程中轻而有节律地施以压力，每日 1～2 次，每次 20 分钟。

3. 拍打及捏筋法

术者在胃压痛点的对侧，后背压痛点处，用拇指轻揉 3～5 分钟，再用四指轻揉剑突下 3～5 分钟，然后环状拍打背压痛点 3～5 分钟。有恶心

on the back in a circle for 3 – 5 minutes. If the patient has nausea, vomiting, and acid regurgitation, after the gently kneading below the xiphous process for 3 – 5 minutes, knead gently, up to down, along the first line of bladder channels on the back by thumb for 3 – 5 minutes and then pat the posterior midline, the left oblique line, and the right oblique line 3 – 5 minutes respectively.

Section Five   Physical exercise

Based on the personal health condition, the patient can perform the whole style or part of Taiji. The patient can also exercise Wuqinxi, Baduanjin, or Baojiancao.

Section Six   Herbal dietary treatment

1. Baikouren 15 g, grain powder 100 g, ferment 50 g (or the same ratio of these three materials).

Get rid of the waste from Baikouren and crush it into fine powder. Scatter it in the fermented powder and make it into regular bun. It helps appetite, fortify the spleen, disperse the food, and eliminate the distention. It is used for chronic gastritis with devitalized appetite and fullness and distention in the stomach and abdomen.

2. Jasmine 6 g, Shichangpu 6 g, green tea 10 g.

Grind the material into fine powder. Pour in the boiling water. Drink the tea at any time, one packet per

呕吐、泛酸者,用四指轻揉剑突下部
3～5分钟,然后用拇指由上而下轻揉
后背第一侧线3～5分钟,再拍打后背
正中线以及左、右斜线各3～5分钟。

(五) 体育疗法

根据自己的身体状况,可全套练
习太极拳,也可分段练习。或经常作
五禽戏、八段锦、保健操等。

(六) 药膳疗法

1. 以白蔻仁 15 g,面粉 100 g,酵
面 50 g 的比例,将白蔻仁去杂质,打
成细末,待面粉发酵后撒入,按常规
制成馒头。具有开胃健脾、消食除胀
之功。用于慢性胃炎之食欲不振、脘
腹胀满等症。

2. 取茉莉花 6 g,石菖蒲 6 g,青
茶 10 g,共为细末,沸水冲泡,随时饮
用。每日 1 剂。主治慢性胃炎所引

慢性胃炎的中医特色疗法

day. It is for chronic gastritis with distending pain in the stomach and abdomen, and non-transformation of food.

3. Ganjiang 6 g, Gaoliangjiang 10, glutinous rice 60 g.

Clean the Ganjiang and Gaoliangjang in water and make a decoction. Filter the sediment and keep the juice. Make congee, putting the clean glutinous rice in the decoction, in slow fire. Eat the congee with duly a-mount. It is for chronic gastritis in the pattern of spleen-stomach deficiency cold.

4. Huaishanyao 30 g, chestnut 60 g, fresh ginger 4 pieces, Chinese date 5 pieces, glutinous rice 60 g.

Put peeled chestnut, Huaishanyao, fresh ginger, non-pitch Chinese date, and cleaned glutinous rice in a pot. Pour duly amount of water and make congee in slow fire. Add some flavoring and eat the congee with duly amount. It is for chronic gastritis in the pattern of spleen-stomach qi deficiency.

5. Tender hen (about 750 g), Huangjing 60 g, Dang-shen 30 g, Huaishanyao 30 g, duly amount of fresh ginger and green onion.

Kill a hen, eliminate the hair and internal organs, clean and cut it into slices. Flavor the chicken with ginger slices, green onion, salt, pepper power, monosodium glutamate, and oil evenly. Clean and crush Huangjing, Dangshen, and Huaishanyao. Evenly mix the hen slices

起的脘腹胀痛、纳谷不化等症。

3. 干姜 6 g,高良姜 10 g,粳米 60 g。将干姜、高良姜洗净,水煎去渣取汁,把粳米洗净,加入药汁中,文火煮成粥,随量食用。适用于脾胃虚寒型的慢性胃炎。

4. 怀山药 30 g,栗子 60 g,生姜 4 片,大枣 5 枚,粳米 60 g。将栗子去皮,大枣去核,与洗净的怀山药、生姜、粳米一齐放入锅内,加清水适量,文火煮成粥,调味随量食用。适用于慢性胃炎属脾胃气虚者。

5. 嫩母鸡 1 只(约 750 g),黄精 60 g,党参 30 g,怀山药 30 g,生姜、葱花各适量。将嫩母鸡活宰,去毛、内脏,洗净,斩块,并用姜丝、葱花、食盐、川椒粉、味精、生油调匀;黄精、党参、怀山药洗净,切碎。把调好味的鸡块与上药共放入碟中,拌匀,放入锅内,隔水蒸熟即可。随量食用。适

慢性胃炎的中医特色疗法

with the herbs in the plate. Steam the hen slices in the pot, separated by the water, to well done. Eat the chicken with duly amount. It is for chronic gastritis in the pattern of spleen-stomach deficiency and weakness.

6. Pig's stomach (about 500 g), Zhike 12 g, Qingpi 6 g, fresh ginger 4 pieces.

Eliminate the fat from the pig's stomach and scratch it with salt. Wash it several times in the water until clean. Soak it in the boiling water to get rid of the stinky odor. Peel the white membrane. Clean Zhike, Chenpi, and fresh ginger. Cook all the stuff in the pot with duly amount of water in high heat. Shift to slow fire for 2 hours after water is boiling. Add the flavoring before done. Drink the soup and eat the chicken with duly amount. It is for chronic gastritis in the pattern of qi stagnation in the liver and stomach.

7. Mutton 250 g, Ganjiang 15 g, Jineijin 12 g, Chinese date 4 pieces.

Clean the mutton and cut it into slices. Stir-fry the mutton in the pot until dry. Clean Ganjiang, Jineijin, and Chinese date(without pitch). Put all the stuff in a pot with duly amount of water. Cook it in a low gas for 1 - 2 hours after water is boiling. Add the flavoring. Drink the soup and eat the mutton with duly amount. It is for chronic gastritis in the pattern of spleen-stomach deficiency cold.

用于慢性胃炎属脾胃虚弱者。

6. 猪肚 1 个(约 500 g),枳壳 12 g,青皮 6 g,生姜 4 片。将猪肚切去肥油,用盐擦洗,并用清水反复漂洗干净,再放入开水中去腥味,刮去白膜;枳壳、陈皮、生姜洗净,把全部用料一齐放入锅内,加清水适量,用武火煮沸后,文火煮 2 小时,调味即可。随量食肉饮汤。适用于慢性胃炎属肝胃气滞者。

7. 羊肉 250 g,干姜 15 g,鸡内金 12 g,大枣 4 枚。将羊肉洗净,切块,并放入锅内炒干水分,干姜、鸡内金、大枣(去核)洗净,一齐放入锅内,加清水适量,武火煮沸后,改文火煮 1～2 小时,调味即可。随量饮汤食肉。适用于慢性浅表性胃炎属脾胃虚寒者。

慢性胃炎的中医特色疗法

8. Sharen 6 g (crush and post-decoct), Foshou 12 g.

Boil Foshou in the water and then add Sharen. Eliminate the sediment and drink the decoction. It is for chronic gastritis in the pattern of binding depression of liver qi.

9. Danshen 15 g, Tanxiang 6 g (decoct later), Sharen 6 g (decoct later).

Boil Danshen in the water and then add Tanxiang and Sharen. Eliminate the sediment and drink the decoction. It is for the chronic gastritis in the pattern of qi stagnation and blood stasis.

10. Shidi 6 g, Dingxiang 6 g, fresh ginger 5 pieces.

Decoct the herbs in water. It is for the chronic gastritis in the pattern of stomach cold.

Chapter Two   The Treatment of Chronic Atrophic Gastritis

Section One   Internal treatment

1. Treatment based on pattern differentiation

(1) Damp-heat in spleen and stomach

Symptoms and signs: Glomus distention or distending pain in the stomach duct, no desire to eat, bitter taste and sticky sensation in the mouth, heavy cumbersome head and body, ungratified defecation, burning feverish

8. 砂仁 6 g(打碎,后下),佛手 12 g。先水煎佛手,后下砂仁,去渣内服。用于慢性胃炎属肝郁气滞者。

9. 丹参 15 g,檀香 6 g(后下),砂仁 6 g(后下)。丹参用水先煎,檀香、砂仁后下,去渣内服。适用于慢性胃炎属气滞血瘀者。

10. 柿蒂 6 g,丁香 6 g,生姜 5 片。水煎服。适用于慢性胃炎属胃寒者。

二、慢性萎缩性胃炎的治疗

(一) 内治疗法

1. 辨证治疗

(1) 脾胃湿热

【证候】 胃脘痞满或胀痛,不思饮食,口苦口黏,头身困重,大便不爽,肛门灼热,舌边尖红、苔黄腻,脉弦滑。

sensation in the anus, red at the tip and the sides of the tongue, yellow slimy fur, and slippery string-like pulse.

Therapeutic methods: Clearing away heat, draining turbidity, harmonizing the stomach and eliminating glomus.

Recipes and herbs: Modified Sanren Decoction includes Baikouren, Yiyiren, Houpo, Banxia, Tongcao, Huashi, Zhuye, Huanglian, Yinchen and Danshen. Supplement Zhuru and Shengjiang to harmonize the stomach and downbear the counterflow for nausea and vomiting. Supplement Zhuru, Huanglian and Zhizi to clear heat, and transform dampness for bitter taste in the mouth, oppression in the chest and yellow slimy fur resulting from the depression of phlegm-damp transforming into the heat. Supplement Dangshen and Fuling to fortify the spleen and disinhibit dampness for stomachache, diarrhea, and fatigue resulting from the qi deficiency failing to transform dampness. Supplement Gualou, and Zhishi to transform phlegm and abduct the stagnation for phlegm stagnation and constipation. Supplement Danshen, Chuanxiong, Sanleng and Ezhu for enduring stasis entering the network vessels. Supplement Xiangru to resolve the exterior and transform dampness for the accompanying of exterior dampness. Supplement Jineijin, Shenqu and Maiya to disperse the food and abduct the stagnation for evident

【治法】 清热泄浊,和胃除痞。

【方药】 三仁汤加减,药用白蔻仁、薏苡仁、厚朴、半夏、通草、滑石、竹叶、黄连、茵陈、丹参。恶心呕吐者,加竹茹、生姜和胃降逆;口苦胸闷、舌苔黄腻者,为痰湿郁而化热,加竹茹、黄连、栀子以清热化湿;胃痛泄泻、倦怠者,为气虚不能化湿,当加入党参、茯苓健脾利湿;痰滞便闭者,加瓜蒌、枳实以化痰导滞;病久入络有瘀者,加丹参、川芎、三棱、莪术等;兼表湿者,加香薷以解表化湿;食欲不振明显者,加鸡内金、神曲、麦芽以消食导滞。

devitalized appetite.

(2) Disharmony of the liver and stomach

Symptoms and signs: Distending and full in the stomach, attacking pain in the stomach duct, pain referring to the rib-sides, oppression in the chest, belching, likeliness to sign, vomiting, vexation, irascibility, dizziness, unpeaceful sleep, inhibited defecation, sloppy diarrhea or constipation, pale red tongue, thin yellow or white fur, string-like pulse.

Therapeutic methods: Soothing the liver, regulating qi, harmonizing the stomach and stopping pain.

Recipes and herbs: Modified Chaihu Shugan Powder includes Chaihu, Zhike, Zhixiangfu, Chuangxiong, Guangchenpi, Shengbaishaoyao, Shenggancao, Honghua, Jingtaoren, Zidanshen and Ezhu. Supplement Yanhusuo, Chuanlianzi and Foshou to reinforce the function of rectifying qi, resolving depression and stopping pain for the evident pain. Supplement Baidoukou, Chenxiang and Xuanfuhua to smooth the counterflow qi for belching. Supplement Mudanpi, Zhizi and Zuojin Wan (pill) for enduring binding depression of liver qi transforming into fire resulting in the depressed fire in the liver and stomach with the presence of burning pain in the stomach, clamoring stomach and acid regurgitation. Supplement Shengdihuang and Mudanpi for liver fire damaging

（2）肝胃不和

【证候】 胃脘胀满攻撑作痛，痛连两胁，胸闷嗳气，善太息，呕哕，心烦易怒，头昏寐差，大便不畅，或便溏，或便秘，舌质淡红、苔薄黄或薄白，脉弦。

【治法】 疏肝理气，和胃止痛。

【方药】 柴胡疏肝散加减。药用柴胡、枳壳、制香附、川芎、广陈皮、生白芍药、生甘草、红花、净桃仁、紫丹参、莪术等。痛甚者，加延胡索、川楝子、佛手，以增强理气解郁止痛之功；嗳气者，加白豆蔻、沉香、旋覆花，以顺气降逆；肝气郁结日久化火，肝胃郁热，胃脘灼痛、嘈杂泛酸者，加牡丹皮、栀子合左金丸；肝火伤阴者，加生地黄、牡丹皮；肝郁气滞血瘀者，加丹参、当归、红花等。

yin. Supplement Danshen, Danggui and Honghua for liver depression, qi stagnation and blood stasis.

(3) Blood stasis obstructing the collaterals

Symptoms and signs: Fixed stabbing or splitting pain in the stomach duct, aggravation after pressure, or vomiting of blood, bloody stool, dark facial complexion, dark purple tongue or with static patches, rough pulse.

Therapeutic methods: Activating blood to remove stasis, freeing the collaterals and relieving pain.

Recipes and herbs: Modified Shixiao Powder includes Puhuang, Wulingzhi, Yanhusuo, Dilong and Qingpi. Supplement Huangqi, Huangjing, Baizhu and Dangshen to boost qi for the accompanying with qi deficiency. Supplement Taoren, Honghua and Chishaoyao to reinforce blood quickening and stasis transformation for the drastic pain resulting from the blood stasis and qi stagnation.

(4) Qi deficiency in the spleen and stomach

Symptoms and signs: Glomus distention in the stomach duct, elusive distending sensation, fullness and obstruction in the stomach duct after eating, fatigue and lack of strength, pale enlarged tongue, thin white fur and deep weak pulse.

Therapeutic methods: Tonifying the spleen and stomach to boost qi.

Recipes and herbs: Modified Buzhong Yiqi Decoc-

（3）瘀血阻络

【证候】 胃脘刺痛或刀割样痛，痛处固定，拒按，或见吐血、黑便、面色晦暗，舌质紫暗或有瘀斑，脉涩。

【治法】 活血化瘀，通络止痛。

【方药】 失笑散加味。药用蒲黄、五灵脂、延胡索、地龙、青皮等。兼有气虚者，加黄芪、黄精、白术、党参以益气；血瘀气滞，疼痛剧者，可加桃仁、红花、赤芍药等，以增强活血化瘀之功。

（4）脾胃气虚

【证候】 胃脘痞闷，似胀非胀，食少纳呆，食后胃脘发堵，倦怠乏力，舌质胖淡、苔薄白，脉沉弱。

【治法】 补中益气。

【方药】 补中益气汤加减。药

tion includes Dangshen, Huangqi, Baizhu, Danggui, Chenpi, Shenggancao, Shengma, Chaihu and Sharen. Supplement Laifuzi and Maiya to disperse food and abduct stagnation for the accompanying with food stagnation. Supplement Gouqizi to boost qi and supplement blood for dual deficiency of qi and blood. Supplement Shensanqi and Baiji to transform the stasis and stanch the bleeding for the accompanying with bleeding.

(5) Deficiency cold in the spleen and stomach

Symptoms and signs: Dull pain, preferring to warmth and pressure, pain alleviated with intake of food, sometimes vomiting of clear water, reduced intake of food, low-spiritedness and fatigue, lack warmth of hands and feet, pale tongue, thin white fur and fine weak pulse.

Therapeutic methods: Boosting qi, warming the middle jiao and invigorating the spleen.

Recipes and herbs: Modified Huangqi Jianzhong Decoction includes Huangqi, Chuanguizhi, Shengshaoyao, Shenggancao, Shengjiang, Dazao, and Yitang. Supplement Chenpi, Banxia and Fuling to downbear the counterflow, harmonize the stomach, fortify the spleen and dry the dampness for profuse vomiting of clear water. Supplement Gaoliangjiang and Xiangfu to reinforce warming the spleen and stomach, dissipating cold and

用党参、黄芪、白术、当归、陈皮、生甘草、升麻、柴胡、砂仁等。挟食滞者，加莱菔子、麦芽等以消食导滞；气血两虚者，加枸杞子以益气补血；兼出血者，加参三七、白及以化瘀止血。

(5) 脾胃虚寒

【证候】 胃脘隐隐作痛，绵绵不断，喜暖喜按，得食则减，时吐清水，纳少，神疲乏力，手足欠温，大便溏薄，舌质淡、苔薄白，脉细弱。

【治法】 益气温中健脾。

【方药】 黄芪建中汤加减。药用黄芪、川桂枝、生芍药、生甘草、生姜、大枣、饴糖等。泛吐清水较多者，加陈皮、半夏、茯苓以降逆和胃，健脾燥湿；胃寒痛甚者，加高良姜、香附，以增强温中散寒止痛之效，痛止后，可服用六君子丸或香砂六君子丸以温健脾胃，巩固疗效；若久痛不止，瘀

relieving pain for drastic cold stomachache. Go on the administration of Liujunzi Pill or Xiangsha Liujunzi Pill to warm and fortify the stomach and spleen to solidify the effect when pain stops. Supplement Honghua, Puhuang, Wulingzhi and Danshen for static blood obstructing the network vessels. Supplement Ganjiangtan, Fulonggan, Baiji and Diyutan for bloody stool.

(6) **Yin deficiency of the spleen and stomach**

Symptoms and signs: Dull burning pain in the stomach duct, vexation, thirst with desire to drink water, burning sensation of clamoring stomach, dry bound stool, dizzy head, poor sleep, reduced intake of food, or feverish sensation in the soles of the hands and feet, red tongue with scanty fur or with fissures on the tongue, or peeling fur and fine rapid pulse.

Therapeutic methods: Nourishing yin, clearing away heat, boosting the stomach and engendering fluid.

Recipes and herbs: Modified Yiwei Decoction includes Shashen, Maimendong, Shengdihuang, Yuzhu, Chaihu, and Digupi. Supplement Huanglian and Zhuye to reinforce draining the heat for severe stomach heat. Supplement a small dose of Chenpi, Shenqu and Maiya to support the smooth downbearing of the stomach qi for poor intake of food. Supplement Shaoyao and Gancao to emolliate the liver, relax tension, and relieve pain for ev-

血阻络者,可加红花、蒲黄、五灵脂、
丹参;便黑者,加干姜炭、伏龙肝、白
及、地榆炭等。

(6)脾胃阴虚

【证候】 胃脘隐隐灼痛,烦渴思
饮,口干咽燥,胃中嘈杂灼热,大便干
结,头昏寐差,食少纳呆,或有手足心
热,舌红少苔或有裂纹,或花剥苔,脉
细数。

【治法】 养阴清热,益胃生津。

【方药】 益胃汤加减。药用沙
参、麦门冬、生地黄、玉竹、柴胡、地骨
皮等。胃热偏重者,加黄连、竹叶以
增泄热之功;纳差者,可少加陈皮、神
曲、麦芽之类以助胃气通降;疼痛较
甚者,可加芍药、甘草以柔肝缓急止
痛;兼有瘀滞者,加丹参、桃仁活血
化瘀。

ident pain. Supplement Danshen and Taoren to quicken the blood and transform the stasis for the accompanying with the stasis and stagnation.

2. Chinese patent medicines

(1) Shanzha Pill

Ingredients: Shanzha, Maiya and Liushenqu.

Functions: Improve appetite and disperse the food.

Indications: Indigestion, collection and stagnation of food, abdominal fullness and distention

Direction: Take one pill processed by honey per time. Take 6 - 8 tablets per time and twice a day. Take 1 packet granule per time and thrice a day.

(2) Zhaqu Pill

Ingredients: Shanzha, Shenqu, Binglang, Shanyao, Baibiandou, Jineijin, Zhike, Maiya and Sharen.

Functions: Harmonizing the stomach and dispersing food.

Indications: Pattern of accumulation and stagnation of food.

Direction: Take 1 pill per time and twice a day.

(3) Xiangsha Pingwei Pill

Ingredients: Muxiang, Chenpi, Sharen, Cangzhu, Gancao, Shengjiang, Houpo and Dazao, etc.

Functions: Regulating qi, harmonizing the stomach,

2. 中成药

(1) 山楂丸

【组成】 山楂、麦芽、六神曲。

【功效】 开胃消食。

【适应证】 消化不良,饮食停滞,脘腹胀满。

【用法】 蜜丸每次 1 丸;片剂每次 6~8 片,每日 2 次;冲剂每次 1 袋,每日 3 次。

(2) 楂曲丸

【组成】 山楂、神曲、槟榔、山药、白扁豆、鸡内金、枳壳、麦芽、砂仁。

【功效】 和胃消食。

【适应证】 饮食积滞之证。

【用法】 每次 1 丸,每日 2 次。

(3) 香砂平胃丸

【组成】 木香、陈皮、砂仁、苍术、甘草、生姜、厚朴、大枣等。

【功效】 理气和胃,燥湿健脾。

drying the dampness and invigorating the spleen.

Indications: Disharmony between the liver and stomach leading to fullness and distention in the abdomen, belching, acid regurgitation, vomiting and sloppy stool.

Direction: Take pill 6 g per time and twice a day.

(4) Shugan Liqi Pill

Ingredients: Houpo, Zhishi, Baishaoyao, Yanhusuo, Xiangfu, Chuanxiong, Chenxiang, Mudanpi, Chaihu, Sharen, Muxiang, Baidoukou and Gancao.

Functions: Soothing the liver, regulating qi, harmonizing the stomach and relieving pain.

Indications: Stagnation of liver qi and disharmony of stomach qi leading to stomachache, poor appetite, nausea and vomiting.

Direction: Take 1 pill per time and twice a day.

(5) Yiwei Paste

Ingredients: Baishaoyao, Muxiang, Chenpi and Gancao, etc.

Functions: Regulating qi, harmonizing the stomach, alleviating pain.

Indications: Stagnation of liver qi leading to stomachache, belching, abdominal distention and poor appetite.

Direction: Take 6 g per time and twice a day.

【适应证】 肝胃不和,脘腹胀满,嗳气吞酸,呕吐便溏等。

【用法】 每次6g,每日2次。

(4) 舒肝理气丸

【组成】 厚朴、枳实、白芍药、延胡索、香附、川芎、沉香、牡丹皮、柴胡、砂仁、木香、白豆蔻、甘草。

【功效】 疏肝理气,和胃止痛。

【适应证】 肝气郁结,胃气不和引起的胃痛、纳差、恶心呕吐等。

【用法】 每次1丸,每日2次。

(5) 益胃膏

【组成】 白芍药、木香、陈皮、甘草等。

【功效】 理气和胃,缓急止痛。

【适应证】 肝郁气滞引起的胃痛、嗳气、腹胀、纳差等。

【用法】 每次6g,每日2次。

(6) Weiling Granule

Ingredients: Awei, Jineijin, Yanhusuo, Xiangfu, Haipiaoxiao, Caojueming and Guangmuxiang, etc.

Functions: Soothing the liver, regulating qi, activating the blood to remove the stasis.

Indications: Liver depression, qi stagnation, and disharmony between the spleen and the stomach leading to stomachache, belching, abdominal distention, and non-transformation of food.

Direction: Take 6 g per time and twice a day.

(7) Jianwei Tablet

Ingredients: Laifuzi, Chaihu, Wulingzhi, Baishaoyao, Cangzhu, Chenpi, Ganjiang, Yanhusuo, Gancao, Chuanlianzi and Caodoukou, etc.

Functions: Regulating qi, relieving pain, harmonizing the stomach and checking the acid.

Indications: Disharmony of the liver and the stomach leading to distending pain in the stomach, belching, and acid regurgitation.

Direction: Take 1.5 g per time and four times a day.

(8) Zuojin Pill

Ingredients: Huanglian and Wuzhuyu.

Functions: Clearing the liver, purging fire, harmonizing the stomach and relieving pain.

Indications: Liver fire assailing the stomach leading

（6）胃灵冲剂

【组成】 阿魏、鸡内金、延胡索、香附、海螵蛸、草决明、广木香等。

【功效】 疏肝理气，活血化瘀。

【适应证】 肝郁气滞，脾胃不和引起的胃痛、吐酸、腹胀、饮食不化等。

【用法】 每次 6 g，每日 2 次。

（7）健胃片

【组成】 莱菔子、柴胡、五灵脂、白芍药、苍术、陈皮、干姜、延胡索、甘草、川楝子、草豆蔻等。

【功效】 理气止痛，和胃制酸。

【适应证】 肝胃不和引起的胃脘胀痛、嗳气、吞酸等。

【用法】 每次 1.5 g，每日 4 次。

（8）左金丸

【组成】 黄连、吴茱萸。

【功效】 清肝泻火，和胃止痛。

【适应证】 肝火犯胃所致的脘

to pain in the stomach and rib-sides, clamoring stomach, bitter taste in the mouth, upflow nausea, and vomiting.

Direction: Take 3 – 6 g per time and twice a day.

(9) Fufang Yanhu Zhitong Tablet

Ingredients: Yanhusuo, Chuanlianzi, Xiangfu and Xuchangqing, etc.

Functions: Regulating qi, activating the blood and relieving pain.

Indications: Disharmony of the liver and the stomach, depressed stagnation of qi and blood leading to gastric pain.

Direction: Take 2 – 4 tablets per time and three times a day.

(10) Wei'an Capsule

Ingredients: Shihu, Baishaoyao, Nanshashen and Huangbai, etc.

Functions: Nourishing yin, boosting the stomach, moving qi, and relieving pain.

Indications: Stomach yin deficiency leading to gastric pain, dry mouth and dry throat, etc.

Direction: Take 6 – 8 capsules per time and three times a week.

(11) Fuzi Lizhong Pill

Ingredients: Zhifuzi, Dangshen, Ganjiang, Baizhu and Gancao.

Functions: Warming and supplementing the spleen

胁疼痛、嘈杂、口苦、泛恶呕吐等。

【用法】 每次3～6g,每日2次。

（9）复方延胡止痛片

【组成】 延胡索、川楝子、香附、徐长卿等。

【功效】 理气活血止痛。

【适应证】 肝胃不和,气血郁滞引起的胃脘痛。

【用法】 每次2～4片,每日3次。

（10）胃安胶囊

【组成】 石斛、白芍药、南沙参、黄柏等。

【功效】 养阴益胃,行气止痛。

【适应证】 胃阴亏虚所致的胃脘疼痛,口干咽干等。

【用法】 每次6～8粒,每日3次。

（11）附子理中丸

【组成】 制附子、党参、干姜、白术、甘草。

【功效】 温补脾胃,散寒止痛。

and stomach, dissipating cold and relieving pain.

Indications: Spleen and stomach deficiency cold.

Direction: Take 1 pill per time and twice a day.

(12) Jianpi Pill

Ingredients: Dangshen, Baizhu, Chenpi, Zhishi, Shanzha, Maiya, Shenqu, Biandou, Lianzi, Guya, Baidoukou, Shanyao, Muxiang, Fuling and Banxia.

Functions: Invigorating the spleen, boosting qi, regulating qi and dispersing the food.

Indications: Weakness of the spleen and stomach leading to impaired splenic movement and transformation resulting in the discomfort and pain in the stomach.

Direction: Take 1 large pill or 9 g small pill processed with honey per time and twice a day.

(13) Qipi Pill

Ingredients: Renshen, Baizhu, Shanzha, Fuling, Liushenqu, Maiya, Zexie, Chenpi, Lianzi, Shanyao and Gancao.

Functions: Invigorating the spleen, harmonizing the stomach and relieving food retention.

Indications: Chronic atrophic gastritis in the pattern of spleen-stomach weakness and food stagnation.

Direction: Take 1 pill per time and three times a day.

【适应证】 脾胃虚寒证。

【用法】 每次1丸,每日2次。

(12)健脾丸

【组成】 党参、白术、陈皮、枳实、山楂、麦芽、神曲、扁豆、莲子、谷芽、白豆蔻、山药、木香、茯苓、半夏。

【功效】 健脾益气,理气消食。

【适应证】 脾胃虚弱,运化失健引起的不思饮食,脘痛不适等。

【用法】 每次大蜜丸1丸,小蜜丸9g,每日2次。

(13)启脾丸

【组成】 人参、白术、山楂、茯苓、六神曲、麦芽、泽泻、陈皮、莲子、山药、甘草。

【功效】 健脾和胃消食。

【适应证】 慢性萎缩性胃炎脾胃虚弱,饮食积滞。

【用法】 每次1丸,每日3次。

3. Simple and proved formulae

（1）Huangpu Weiyan Decoction

Ingredients：Shenghuangqi 30 g，Pugongying 20 g，Baihe 20 g，Wuyao 10 g，Baishaoyao 20 g，Gancao 10 g，Danshen 20 g，Chaoshenqu 10 g，Chaoshanzha 10 g，Chaomaiya 10 g.

Functions：Boosting qi，clearing away heat，invigorating the spleen and harmonizing the stomach.

Indications：Chronic atrophic gastritis in the pattern of spleen-stomach weakness leading to food stagnation and internal depressed heat.

Direction：Decoct the herbs in water. Take one packet a day.

（2）Sanwei Powder

Ingredients：steamed Shanyao 100 g，raw Jineijin 100 g，Banxia 60 g（processed with vinegar）.

Functions：Invigorating the spleen and harmonizing the stomach.

Indications：Chronic atrophic gastritis in the pattern of spleen-stomach weakness.

Direction：Grind the herbs into extreme fine powder. Take powder 3 g with warm water prior to each meal every day. Two months consist of one course. Add Zhebeimu 50 g for acid regurgitation. Add Sanqi 20 g, and Baiji 50 g for bleeding.

3. 单方验方

（1）黄蒲胃炎汤

【组成】 生黄芪 30 g,蒲公英 20 g,百合 20 g,乌药 10 g,白芍药 20 g,甘草 10 g,丹参 20 g,炒神曲 10 g,炒山楂 10 g,炒麦芽 10 g。

【功用】 益气清热,健脾和胃。

【适应证】 慢性萎缩性胃炎脾胃虚弱,食滞不化,内有郁热者。

【用法】 水煎服,每日 1 剂。

（2）三味散

【组成】 蒸熟山药 100 g,生鸡内金 100 g,醋制半夏 60 g。

【功用】 健脾和胃。

【适应证】 慢性萎缩性胃炎脾胃虚弱者。

【用法】 上药共研极细末,每日 3 次,每次 3 g,饭前温开水送服,2 个月为 1 个疗程。吞酸者加浙贝母 50 g;出血者加三七 20 g,或白及 50 g。

(3) Shanzha Maiya Decoction

Ingredients: crystal sugar 20 g, Shanzha 50 g, Maiya 25 g.

Functions: Invigorating the stomach and relieving food retention.

Indications: Chronic atrophic gastritis with little acid regurgitation.

Direction: Decoct the herbs in water. Drink the decoction twice a day.

(4) Shanzha Mitang Syrup

Ingredients: crystal sugar 20 g, Shanzha 60 g, honey 30 g.

Functions: Invigorating the stomach, relieving food retention and resolving the stagnation.

Indications: Chronic strophic gastritis with low acid regurgitation.

Direction: Steam the herbs to syrup in the non-iron container. Take 2 - 4 spoons each time after the meal for long-term use.

(5) Yiwei Wumei

Ingredient: Wumeirou.

Functions: Engendering the fluids and astringing.

Indications: Atrophic gastritis with little gastric acid.

Direction: Bake the herb slightly and take it as a

（3）山楂麦芽汤

【组成】 冰糖 20 g，山楂 50 g，麦芽 25 g。

【功用】 健胃消食。

【适应证】 萎缩性胃炎胃酸低者。

【用法】 水煎服，每日 2 次。

（4）山楂蜜糖酱

【组成】 冰糖 20 g，山楂 60 g，蜂蜜 30 g。

【功用】 健胃消食化滞。

【适应证】 萎缩性胃炎胃酸低者。

【用法】 将上药放入非铁器皿中蒸熟如果酱，每次饭后食入 2～4 匙，可长期服用。

（5）一味乌梅

【组成】 乌梅肉。

【功用】 生津收敛。

【适应证】 萎缩性胃炎胃酸低者。

【用法】 乌梅肉略焙。每日作

snack every day.

Section Two   Emotional therapy

The occurrence and development of chronic gastritis is closely related to the emotional changes. Especially for the long-term patient, he will feel anxious and restless, suspecting himself suffering from the cancer. It does no good to the health, but aggravates the condition. So after the excluding the possibility of cancer through the examination, the patient must build up confidence in the triumph over the disease. Keep in a good humor. Cultivate a good mood. Avoid the unfavorable emotional stimulation.

Section Three   Herbal dietary therapies

1. Huangjing 30 g, Dangshen 15 g, Huangqi 15 g, Huaishanyao 30 g, black glutinous rice 60 g. Use all the materials to make congee in duly amount water in the pot in slow fire. Take out Huangqi and add flavoring. Eat with duly amount. It is for chronic atrophic gastritis in the pattern of spleen-stomach weakness.

2. Lean pork 250 g, Baishaoyao 12 g, Shihu 12 g, Chinese date 4 pieces. Clean the lean pork and cut it into slice. Take out the pitches of Chinese dates. After cleaning, boil the sliced lean pork, Baishaoyao, Shihu,

零食吃。

（二）情志疗法

慢性胃炎的发生发展与情志变化关系密切,尤其是病程较久者,常有焦虑不安的恐癌心理,这不仅无益于疾病的治疗,相反会加重病情,使病变进一步恶化。因此在通过检查,排除"癌变"的同时,患者必须树立战胜疾病的信心。平时注意保持愉快的心情,培养良好的情绪,减少不良情绪的刺激。

（三）药膳疗法

1. 黄精 30 g,党参 15 g,黄芪 15 g,怀山药 30 g,黑糯米 60 g,一起放入锅内,加清水适量,文火煮成粥,去黄芪,调味即可。随量食用。适用于慢性萎缩性胃炎脾胃虚弱者。

2. 猪瘦肉 250 g,白芍药 12 g,石斛 12 g,大枣 4 枚。将瘦猪肉洗净切块,白芍药、石斛、大枣(去核)洗净,一齐放入锅内,加清水适量,武火烧

Chinese dates in duly amount water in a pot for 1 - 2 hours. It can be used to treat atrophical gastritis due to yin deficiency.

3. One pig stomach (about 500 g), fresh Foshou 15 g, Yanhusuo 10 g and 4 pieces of ginger. The pig stomach is washed and cooked with other ingredients with strong fire. After it is boiled, it is heated with mild fire for 1 - 2 hours. It can be used to treat atrophical gastritis due to disharmony of the liver and stomach, qi stagnation and blood stasis.

4. One Squid (about 300 g), Shanzha 30 g, Huaishanyao 30 g and some ginger. The squid and other ingredients are washed and cooked together with strong fire. When it is boiled, it is heated with mild fire. It is used to treat atrophical chronic gastritis due to spleen deficiency and food retention.

5. Jinlingzi 10 g and Yanhusuo 10 g are decocted. This decoction can be used to treat chronic gastritis due to liver stagnation and qi stagnation.

6. Jupi 6 g, Daidaihua 6 g and Gancao 3 g are cut

沸后,文火煮1～2小时,调味即可,随量饮汤食肉。适用于慢性萎缩性胃炎阴亏有热者。

3. 猪肚1个(约500 g),鲜佛手15 g,延胡索10 g,生姜4片。将猪肚除去肥油,用盐擦洗,并用清水反复漂洗干净,再放入开水内脱去腥味,刮去白膜;佛手(切片)、延胡索、生姜洗净。一起放入锅内,加清水适量,武火煮沸后,改文火煮1～2小时,调味即可。随量饮汤食肉。适用于慢性萎缩性胃炎肝胃不和,气滞血瘀者。

4. 鲤鱼1条(约300 g),山楂30 g,怀山药30 g,生姜适量。将鲤鱼去鳞、腮及肠脏,洗净,切块,起油锅,用姜爆香后,取出备用;山楂、怀山药洗净。把全部用料一起放入锅内,加清水适量,武火煮沸,文火煮1～2小时,调味即可。随量饮汤食肉。适用于慢性萎缩性胃炎属脾虚食滞者。

5. 金铃子10 g,延胡索10 g,水煎服。适用于慢性胃炎肝郁气滞有热者。

6. 橘皮6 g,玳玳花6 g,甘草

into pieces, soaked in boiled water and drunken frequently. It can be used to treat chronic atrophical gastritis due to stagnation of spleen and stomach Qi.

7. Juice of Shengdihuang 30 ml is decocted with rice. This meal is used to treat chronic atrophical gastritis due to internal heat caused by yin deficiency.

8. Shanyao 60 g is cut into pieces and cooked into porridge. It can be used to treat chronic atrophical gastritis due to weakness of spleen Qi.

Chapter Three   Treatments of the Main Symptoms of Chronic Gastritis

Section One   Gastralgia

Gastralgia is the pain felt in the stomach especially at the epigastric area. From the TCM point of view, it is mainly caused by exogenous evil invasion, irregular dieting habits, emotional factors, stomach and spleen deficiencey, etc.

1. Treatments based on pattern differentiation

(1) Cold evil in the stomach

Symptoms and signs: A sudden onset of severe gastric pain, dislike of cold, preference to warmth, but aggravated by cold. No thirst, and preference to hot drinks

3 g,三味药切碎,用滚水泡,不拘时饮服。适用于慢性萎缩性胃炎脾胃气滞者。

7. 生地黄汁 30 ml,如常法煮白米粥,粥临熟时入地黄汁,搅匀食之。适用于慢性萎缩性胃炎阴虚内热者。

8. 山药 60 g,切碎煮粥,一日分服。用于慢性萎缩性胃炎脾虚气弱者。

三、慢性胃炎主症的治疗

(一)胃痛

胃痛是指上腹胃脘部近心窝处经常发生疼痛的一种症状表现。中医学认为,其发生多与外邪侵袭、情志不调或饮食不节、脾胃虚弱等因素有关。

1. 辨证治疗

(1)寒邪客胃

【证候】 胃痛暴作,恶寒喜暖,得温则痛减,遇寒则痛增,口和不渴,喜热饮,苔薄白,脉弦紧。

when drinking. Thin and white tongue coating and the taut pulse.

Therapeutic methods: Dispersing cold in the stomach and stopping pain.

Recipes and herbs: If the pain is mild, just drink ginger and brown sugar decoction, or place a hot water bottle onto the epigastria area, the pain will stop. If the pain is moderate or severe, use "Liangfu Pill" formula plus other herbs such as Gaoliangjiang, Xiangfu, Zisu, Jingjiesui, Biba, Shengjiang and Houpo, etc. If the pain is caused by wind-cold with symptoms such as aversion to cold, fever, headache and general pain, add Fangfeng, Qianghuo, Duhuo, Douchi to strengthen the effect of dispelling wind-cold. If the cold has stagnated too long inside the stomach and transformed into heat or the cold evil is still there, add Huanglian, Wuzhuyu, Zhibanxia and Ganjiang to clear away heat and dispel the cold evil. If the pain is caused by cold and the retention of food, herbs like Zhishi, Dahuang, Jiaosanxian and Jineijin can be added to relieve food stagnation.

(2) Food retention in the stomach

Symptoms and signs: Epigastric pain, abdominal distension, acid regurgitation, vomiting of undigested food, belching with putrid odour and unsmooth movement of bowel, thick and greasy tongue coating with a slippery

【治法】 散寒止痛。

【方药】 轻症可用局部温熨,或服生姜红糖汤即可止痛。较重者可用良附丸加味。药用高良姜、香附、紫苏、荆芥穗、荜茇、生姜、厚朴等。若兼见恶寒、发热、头痛身痛等风寒表证者,加防风、羌活、独活、豆豉等以加强疏风散寒解表的作用;若寒郁化热而寒邪未尽者,可加黄连、吴茱萸、制半夏、干姜以辛散郁热,温化寒邪;若寒挟食滞者,宜加枳实、大黄、焦三仙、鸡内金等以消食导滞。

(2) 饮食停滞

【证候】 胃脘疼痛,胀满,嗳腐吞酸,或呕吐不消化食物,吐食或矢气后痛减,或大便不爽,苔厚腻,脉滑。

pulse.

Therapeutic methods: Removing food retention and promoting digestion.

Recipes and herbs: Modified Zhishi Daozhi Wan. Ingredients: Zhishi, Laifuzi, Dahuang, Jiaosanxian, Jineijin, Houpo and Banxiaqu, etc. If the retention of food is accompanied with slight fever and dislike of cold, add Jinyinhua, Lianqiao, Zisuye and Jingjiesui to release exogenous evils. If the patient belches a lot, regurgitates and even vomits out undigested food, add Chenpi, Shengjiang, Jiangbanxia and Xuanfuhua, etc. to calm the rebellious stomach qi and stop vomiting. If the food retention is caused by accumulated heat in the stomach, herbs such as Lianqiao and Huanglian can be added into the formula to clear away the accumulated heat in the stomach.

(3) Liver qi invading the stomach

Symptoms and signs: Abdominal distension, hypochondriac pain or pain in the whole middle Jiao, frequent belching, unsmooth movement of bowel and emotional factors which exacerbate the pain, thin and white tongue coating and the pulse is deep wiry or taut.

Therapeutic methods: Soothing the liver and regulating qi.

Recipes and herbs: Modified Sini Powder and

【治法】 消食导滞。

【方药】 枳实导滞丸加减。药用枳实、莱菔子、大黄、焦三仙、鸡内金、厚朴、半夏曲等。若停食着凉兼恶寒发热者,加金银花、连翘、紫苏叶、荆芥穗以疏解表邪;兼胃气逆而呕恶呃逆者,加橘皮、生姜、姜半夏、旋覆花等以降逆止呕;兼食积郁热者,加连翘、黄连等以清泻胃肠之热。

(3) 肝气犯胃

【证候】 胃脘胀闷,攻撑作痛,脘痛连胁,嗳气频繁,大便不畅,每因情志因素而痛作,苔多薄白,脉沉弦。

【治法】 疏肝理气。

【方药】 四逆散合金铃子散加

Jinlingzi Powder. Ingredients: Chaihu (prepared with vinegar), Baishaoyao (fry with vinegar), Zhike and Yanhusuo, etc. If liver qi is stagnated and has been transformed into heat which has affected the stomach, and having acid regurgitation, herbs that can clear away heat such as Mudanpi, Zhizi and Huanglian are added. If there is disharmony between the liver and the spleen which leads to liver being depressed, and together with spleen deficiency, causing poor appetite, abdominal and hypochondriac distension, add Taizishen, Houpo and Chenpi, etc. to sooth the liver, nourish and strengthen the spleen. For patients who belch a lot, add Xuanfuhua, Daizheshi, Daodouzi and Chenxiang, etc. to redirect the rebellious qi downwards. If acid regurgitation is accompanied herbs that can neutralize or absorb hydrochloric acid, such as Wuzeigu, Walengzi (calcined), Muli (calcined) and Wulingzhi can be added.

(4) Liver fire causing stomach heat

Symptoms and signs: Epigastric pain, stress or emotional upset aggravates the pain, easiness to get irritated, acid regurgitation, borborygmus, dry mouth with bitter taste, red tongue with yellow coating and pulse is rapid and wiry.

Therapeutic methods: Soothing the liver, clearing away stomach heat and harmonizing the stomach.

减。药用醋柴胡、醋炒白芍药、枳壳、甘草、延胡索、炒川楝子等。若肝郁化热,胃部灼热,嘈杂反酸者,加牡丹皮、栀子、黄连以清泻肝胃之热;兼见肝郁脾虚,不思饮食,脘胁胀满者,加太子参、厚朴、陈皮等以健脾舒肝;嗳气呃逆者,加旋覆花、代赭石、刀豆子、沉香等以顺气降逆;胃酸多者,加乌贼骨、煅瓦楞子、煅牡蛎、五灵脂等以和胃制酸。

(4) 肝胃郁热

【证候】 胃脘疼痛,痛势急迫,烦躁易怒,泛酸嘈杂,口干口苦,舌红苔黄,脉弦或数。

【治法】 疏肝泄热和胃。

Recipes and herbs: Use Huagan Decoction as the basic formula. Ingredients: Qingpi, Chenpi, Shaoyao, Mudanpi, Zhizi, Zixie and Beimu, etc.

(5) Damp-heat stagnating in the stomach

Symptoms and signs: Epigastric pain with hot sensations, abdominal distension, bitter taste with sticky mouth, heavy head and body sensation, poor appetite, borborygmus, difficulty in defecation, accompanied with sore anus, dysuria, yellow greasy tongue coating, and the slippery and rapid pulse.

Therapeutic methods: Resolving and clearing damp heat, regulating qi and harmonizing the stomach.

Recipes and herbs: Modified Lianpo Decoction and Liuyi Powder. Ingredients: Wuzhuyu and Huoxiang. For patients with more heat than dampness, add Huangqin and Dahuang to purge fire and clear away heat. If the dampness is severe, add Yiyiren, Peilan, and Heyin to strengthen the effect of resolving dampness. If the liver fire is turning into heat in stomach and causing gastric bleeding, add Xijiao, Shengdihuang, Mudanpi, Dahuang and Sanqi, etc. to clear away the heat, cool down blood and stop bleeding.

(6) Gastric blood stasis

Symptoms and signs: Gastric pain and the pain is normally fixed with prickling sensation at an area of the

【方药】 化肝煎为主方。药用青皮、陈皮、芍药、牡丹皮、栀子、泽泻、贝母等。

（5）湿热阻胃

【证候】 胃脘热痛，胸脘痞满，口苦口黏，头身重着，纳呆嘈杂，肛门灼热，大便不爽，小便不利，舌苔黄腻，脉滑数。

【治法】 清化湿热，理气和胃。

【方药】 连朴饮合六一散加减。药用黄连、厚朴、栀子、清半夏、吴茱萸、藿香、六一散。偏热者，加黄芩、大黄以加强清热泻火之力；偏湿者，加薏苡仁、佩兰、荷叶以增强芳香化湿之力；若见肝胃郁热，迫血妄行者，加犀角、生地黄、牡丹皮、大黄、三七等清热凉血止血之品。

（6）瘀血停滞

【证候】 胃脘疼痛，痛有定处而拒按，或痛有针刺感，食后痛甚，或见

abdomen. Pressing aggravates the pain and it gets worse after meal. Some patients even vomit blood or have very black stools. The tongue proper is often dark purple and the pulse is sluggish and uneven.

Therapeutic methods: Regulating qi to relieve stagnation, activating blood to remove blood stasis.

Recipes and herbs: Modified Shixiao Powder and Danshen Decoction. Ingredients: Shengpuhuang, Wulinzi, Shengdahuang, Tanxiang and Sanqi, etc. If there is a symptom of vomiting blood and a red tongue proper with yellow coating together with a rapid and taut pulse, it shows that the liver and the stomach are invaded with heat evil, leading to blood oozing out of its vessels. Therefore, Huangqin, Huanglian, Baimaogen and Mudanpi can be added to purge heat and cool down blood. If the condition is caused by stomach and spleen cold and deficiency, and the spleen fails its function of controlling of blood and shows symptoms of bleeding with dull red colour, sallow facial complexion cold extremities and having a pale tongue proper with weak pulse, add Renshen, Huangqi, Xianhecao and Baicaoshuang, etc. to warm up and nourish the spleen, thereby strengthening spleen qi and controlling and stopping bleeding. If the bleeding is quite severe, add Ejiao, Baiji and Shihuisan to strengthen the effect of stopping bleeding.

吐血便黑,舌质紫黯,脉涩。

【治法】 理气行郁,活血化瘀。

【方药】 失笑散合丹参饮加减。药用丹参、生蒲黄、五灵脂、生大黄、檀香、三七粉等。若呕血伴舌红苔黄,脉弦数者,属肝胃郁热,迫血妄行,加黄芩、黄连、白茅根、牡丹皮等以清热泻火;若出血暗红,面色萎黄,四肢不温,舌淡脉弱者,属脾胃虚寒,脾不统血,宜加人参、黄芪、仙鹤草、百草霜等以温脾益气,统摄止血;出血量多而症状较重者,可加阿胶、白及、十灰散加强止血作用。

(7) Deficiency of stomach yin

Symptoms and signs: Dull pain around epigastic area, dry mouth, sore throat, hard stool, red and dry tongue proper with a thin and rapid pulse.

Therapeutic methods: Nourishing yin and reinforcing the stomach.

Recipes and herbs: Modified Yiwei Tang. Ingredients: Baishashen, Maimendong, Shengdihuang, Yuzhu, Baishaoyao, Tianmendong and Gancao, etc. For patrents with symptoms of acid regurgitation and borborygmus, add Huanglian and a small amount of Wuzhuyu to purge fire in the liver and the gallbladder. For liver fire impairing stomach yin, add Mudanpi, Zhizi and Shihu to clear away liver heat and nourish stomach yin. If the liver fire is excess and has affected kidney yin, add Huangbai, Zhimu, Shudihuang and Zhizi to purge the excess liver fire and nourish liver and kidney yin. For patients with stomach fire and heat, add Shengshigao and Shengdahuang to clear away stomach heat and purge the fire.

(8) Cold and deficiency of the stomach and spleen

Symptoms and signs: Dull epigastric pain, preference to warmth and pressing, empty stomach aggravating the pain, pain receding after meal, regurgitation, poor appetite, lethargic, cold extremities, diarrhoea, pale tongue with white coating and the weak and slow pulse.

（7）胃阴亏虚

【证候】 胃痛隐隐，口燥咽干，大便干结，舌红少津，脉细数。

【治法】 养阴益胃。

【方药】 益胃汤加减。药用北沙参、麦门冬、生地黄、玉竹、白芍药、天门冬、甘草等。兼灼痛嘈杂反酸者，加黄连，少佐吴茱萸以疏泻肝胆郁火；肝火伤阴者，加牡丹皮、栀子、石斛以清肝热而养阴；若肝郁火盛，灼烁肾阴者，加黄柏、知母、熟地黄、栀子以泻肝肾之火，滋肝肾之阴；胃火盛者，加生石膏、生大黄以清胃泻火。

（8）脾胃虚寒

【证候】 胃痛隐隐，喜温喜按，空腹痛甚，得食痛减，泛吐清水，纳差，神疲乏力，甚则手足不温，大便溏薄，舌淡苔白，脉虚弱或迟缓。

Therapeutic methods: Warming and invigorating the spleen.

Recipes and herbs: Huangqi Jianzhong Tang as the basic formula. Ingredients: Huangqi, Dangshen, Guizhi, Baishaoyao, Ganjiang, Gancao and Yanhusuo, etc. For patients with symtoms of regurgitation of clear fluid and drooling of sputum, add Chenpi, Jiangbanxia, Baizhu and Fuling to strengthen the spleen and to resolve phlegm. For symptom of acid regurgitation, add Wuzeigu, calcined Walengzi and Wuzhuyu to relieve constraint in the liver and stop acid regurgitation. If the patient suffers from stomach and spleen cold, remove Guizhi and add Fuzi, Shujiao and Rougui to warm the middle jiao and disperse cold.

2. Simple and proved formulae

(1) Wuzei Beimu Powder

Ingredients: Wuzeigu and Beimu.

Actions: Neutralizing acid.

Indications: Gastralgia and acid regurgitation.

Usage and dosage: Grind these two herbs into powder. Take 3 g with warm water each time.

(2) Xiangfu Liangjiang Decoction

Ingredients: Xiangfu 6 g and Gaoliangjiang 3 g.

Actions: Warming the stomach, regulating qi and dispersing cold.

【治法】 温中健脾。

【方药】 黄芪建中汤为主方。药用黄芪、党参、桂枝、白芍药、干姜、甘草、延胡索等。若兼见泛吐清水痰涎者，加陈皮、姜半夏、白术、茯苓以健脾助运，温化痰饮；兼嘈杂反酸者，加乌贼骨、煅瓦楞子和吴茱萸以暖肝制酸；内寒偏盛者，加附子、蜀椒，去桂枝改用肉桂以加强温中散寒之力。

2. 单方验方

（1）乌贼贝母散

【组成】 乌贼骨、贝母各等份。

【功用】 制酸。

【适应证】 胃脘痛泛酸明显者。

【用法】 共研末，每次服用 3 g。

（2）香附良姜汤

【组成】 香附 6 g，高良姜 3 g。

【功用】 温胃理气散寒。

Indications: Gastralgia caused by cold and qi stagnation.

Usage and dosage: Decoct these two herbs and take once daily.

(3) Qingmuxiang Powder

Ingredients: Qingmuxiang.

Actions: Promoting movement of qi and alleviating pain.

Indications: Gastralgia caused by qi stagnation.

Usage and dosage: Grind into powder and take 3 g with warm water.

(4) Sanqi Baiji Dahuang Powder

Ingredients: Sanqi 3 g, Baiji 4.5 g, and Dahuang powder 1.5 g.

Actions: Activating blood, removing blood stasis and stopping bleeding.

Indications: Gastralgia caused by blood stasis, vomiting blood and bloody stool.

Usage and dosage: Mix Powder of these three herbs together and take 3 g with warm water.

(5) Ganjiang Powder

Ingredients: Ganjiang 50 g and rice soup.

Actions: Warming the middle jiao, dispersing cold and alleviating pain.

Indications: Stomachache and gastralgia caused by

【适应证】　寒凝气滞引起的胃脘痛。

【用法】　煎水服用,每日1剂。

（3）青木香散

【组成】　青木香适量。

【功用】　行气导滞。

【适应证】　气滞型胃脘痛。

【用法】　研细末,每服3g。

（4）三七白及大黄粉

【组成】　三七3g,白及4.5g,大黄粉1.5g。

【功用】　活血化瘀止血。

【适应证】　胃脘痛瘀血证,呕血黑便者。

【用法】　三味均匀混合,每服3g。

（5）干姜末

【组成】　干姜50g,米汤适量。

【功用】　温中散寒止痛。

【适应证】　寒性胃痛。孕妇、阴

cold. Contraindications: Pregnancy, yin deficiency and bleeding caused by heat in blood.

Usage and dosage: Use 50 g dry ginger, soak it into warm water for 10 minutes and take it out from water, cover with a damp flannel for 8 hours. After that, grate the ginger and bake it dry. Once it is dried, grind it into powder. Take 3 g with rice soup twice a day. A small amount of cold water can be taken afterwards.

(6) Jiangzhi Houpo

Ingredients: Houpo 100 g, Shengjiang juice and a bowel of rice soup.

Actions: Regulating the movement of qi, removing stagnation and strengthening the stomach.

Indications: Abdominal distension and stomachache caused by qi stagnation. Contra-indication: Pregnancy.

Usage and dosage: Soak Houpo for a while, and chop it into small pieces, then soak it into ginger juice for 2 hours prior to baking on a low heat till completely dried out. Grind the dried Houpo into powder store it in a airtight container. Take 10 g with a bowl of rice water half hour before meal.

(7) Xiangfu Ruxiang Powder

虚内热、血热妄行者均忌服。

【用法】 首先挑选干姜 50 g,除净杂质,去尽泥沙,再用温开水浸泡 10 分钟,倒入瓷盅或瓷盆内,上用浸透的麻布、白布或毛巾盖紧约 8 小时,取出切片,或切成小块或细末,再经炕干,研为细末备用。另取米汤一大碗备用。每次服用 3 g 药末,用米汤为引服下,每日早晚各 1 次,服后宜适量饮用一些冷开水。

(6) 姜汁厚朴

【组成】 厚朴 100 g,生姜汁少许,米汤 1 大碗。

【功用】 行气导滞健胃。

【适应证】 气滞胃痛,以胀痛为主者。孕妇禁用。

【用法】 厚朴经浸泡后,用刀切为极细小的片,放入生姜汁中浸泡 2 小时,并拌匀,取出药片,经炕干或晒干后,研为极细末,装入玻璃瓶内备用。每次服 10 g,每日 3 次,饭前半小时用米汤吞服为佳。

(7) 香附乳香散

Ingredients: Hongqu, Xiangfu and Ruxiang.

Actions: Regulating qi and activating blood.

Indications: Gastralgia caused by qi and blood stagnation. Contra-indications: Pregnancy.

Usage and dosage: Firstly smash Hongqu into small pieces, and fry dry in wok, and then grind it into a powder. Xiangfu and Ruxiang are also ground into powder. Mix these three herbs powder together and store in a airtight container. Take 10 g of the mixed powder in 15 ml of warm red wine or Chinese yellow wine three time daily after meal. Followed by drinking a small glass of warm water.

(8) Shuihonghuazi Decoction

Ingredients: Shuihonghuazi 30 g and mineral water in a proper amount.

Actions: Activating blood to remove blood stasis.

Indications: Gastralgia caused by qi and blood stagnation.

Usage and dosage: Decoct Shuihonghuazi in a proper amount of mineral water and boil it down with mild fire to approximately half of initial amount of water, and extract 300 ml of the decocted liquid. Take 100 ml 3 times a day, and drink a small glass of cold boiled water afterwards.

【组成】 红曲、香附、乳香各等量,白酒或黄酒各适量。

【功用】 行气活血。

【适应证】 气滞血瘀所致的胃脘痛。孕妇慎用。

【用法】 将红曲打碎,分别装入铁锅内炒干脆后,取出研为粉末,将上三味放在一起拌匀,装入瓶内备用。每次服用 10 g,用温热酒为引药吞服,每日 3 次,服后宜适量饮一些白开水。

(8) 水红花子饮

【组成】 水红花子 30 g,矿泉水适量。

【功用】 活血化瘀。

【适应证】 气滞血瘀引起的胃脘痛。

【用法】 将水红花子放沙锅内,加入适量的矿泉水,浸泡 10 分钟后,用文火煎煮至已加入水的一半为止,取 300 ml 药液待用。每次饮服 300 ml,每日 3 次,服后应随意饮用一些冷开水为佳。

(9) Zhike Shanzha Powder

Ingredients: Zhike 50 g, Shanzha 50 g, Maiya 30 g, Laifuzi 40 g, Jineijin 20 g, Qingpi 15 g and Sanleng 12 g.

Actions: Regulating qi and relieving food stagnation.

Indications: Stomachache and gastralgia caused by food stagnation.

Usage and dosage: Oven dry above herbs in a low heat, then grind them into powder and sieve them again before storing the mixed powder into an airtight glass container. Take 20 g with rice soup twice a day before meals.

3. External therapy

Compress: Warm up 250 g of fine salt and wrap it into a piece of muslin and places onto the painful area of the abdomen.

4. Acupuncture treatment

(1) Body acupuncture

Mainly treat foot jueyin and foot yangming channels if gastralgia is caused by liver qi invading stomach. Points used are Zhongwan (CV 12), Qimen (LR 14), Neiguan (PC 6), Zusanli (ST 36) and Yanglingquan (GB 34), etc. Reducing method should be used. If gastralgia is cansed by empty cold of spleen and stomach use points of

（9）枳壳山楂散

【组成】 枳壳、山楂各 50 g，麦芽 30 g，莱菔子 40 g，鸡内金 20 g，青皮 15 g，三棱 12 g。

【功用】 行气消食化滞。

【适应证】 气滞食积之胃痛。

【用法】 上药经晒干或炕干脆后，研为极细粉末，或过细箩，倒入瓷盘内，经充分拌匀后，装入玻璃瓶内。每次服用 20 g，或装入空心胶囊吞服，用米汤直接吞服为佳。每日服2次。

3. 外治法

熨敷法：食盐适量炒热，趁热敷熨胃痛部位。

4. 针灸疗法

（1）体针

肝气犯胃，取足厥阴、阳明经穴为主，常用中脘、期门、内关、足三里、阳陵泉等穴，毫针刺用泻法；脾胃虚寒，取背俞、任脉经穴为主，常用脾俞、胃俞、中脘、章门、内关、足三里等穴，毫针刺用补法，配合灸治。

Pishu (BL 20), Weishu (BL 21), Zhongwan (CV 12), Zhangmen (LR 13), Neiguan (PC 6) and Zusanli (ST 36), etc. Tonifying method should be used, plus use of moxibustion.

(2) Auricular acupuncture

Choose points of stomach, spleen, Jiaogan, Shenmen and Pizhixia, use 3 – 5 points each time and leave for 30 minutes if using acupuncture needles. If the patient suffers from acid regurgitation use Neifenmi instead of stomach point.

(3) Acupoint injection

Choose point of Weishu (BL 21), Pishu (BL 20) and related Jiaji (Extra), Zhongwan (CV 12), Neiguan (PC 6) and Zusanli (ST 36). Use different injetion accordingly, such as Honghua or Danggui injection liquid, and inject into 1 – 3 points each time.

(4) Cupping

Cupping the upper abdomen and the back immediately after acupuncture treatment. It is particularly benificial to gastralgia caused by deficiency type.

(5) Scraping therapy

Choose conception vessel and urinary bladder channel. Clean the area with 75% surgical spirit from Shangwan (CV 13) to Xiawan (CV 10) and the Back-Shu points which are located on the first tract of urinary bladder channel. Use spoon or a coin to scrape the area 20 –

（2）耳针

选用胃、脾、交感、神门、皮质下，用时取 3～5 穴，留针 30 分钟，或用电针、埋针。泛酸多，去胃加内分泌。

（3）穴位注射

选穴胃俞、脾俞、相应夹脊、中脘、内关、足三里。选用红花注射液、当归注射液、阿托品或普鲁卡因注射液等注射于上述穴位，每次 1～3 穴。

（4）拔罐

选用上腹部和背部穴位拔火罐，在针灸后进行。适用于虚性胃痛。

（5）刮痧疗法

在患者上脘、中脘、下脘部和胸骨柄及脊椎两侧，用 75% 的酒精消毒后，用汤匙或硬币由上往下刮动，重复 20～30 次，用力适度，以皮肤出现紫红色皮下出血点为度。

30 times with moderate strength till the skin becomes purple red colour.

(6) Massage therapy

Using either thumb or thane massage areas of Zhongwan (CV 12), Neiguan (PC 6), Zusanli (ST 36) and Zhiyang (GV 9) points. The pressure should start from light, then gradually moderate to heavy and check the pressure with the patient till it is comfortable for him /her. Massage the areas till pain is subsided and then press point for 5 minutes. Massage is good for treating dull pain of the abdomen.

Section Two　Feeling of fullness and oppression

It is a symptom due to sluggish flow of stomach qi. Patients often feel uncomfortable around epigastric area, and the area is soft on touch and no pain on palpating. This condition is often caused by phlegm knotted with qi, food stagnation, damp heat in the middle jiao, emotional or mental imbalance, spleen and stomach qi deficiency, wrong medicine being taken and deficiency of zhenqi and the sluggish spleen's transporting and transforming function leading to dysfunction of stomach and imbalance of stomach qi transforming.

1. Treatment according to syndrome differentiation

(1) Evil heat accumulating in the body

（6）按摩

用拇指在患者中脘穴、内关穴、足三里穴和至阳穴重压揉按，用力由轻至重，由重到轻，直至胃脘痛缓解后再按压 5 分钟。适用于胃脘痛诸证。

（二）痞满

痞满是指胃脘部闭塞不通，胸膈满闷不舒，外无胀急之形，触之濡软，按之不痛的证候。多因痰气搏结，饮食阻滞，湿热中阻，情志失和，脾胃虚弱，误下伤中，正虚邪陷等多种原因导致脾失健运，胃失和降，气机升降失常而成。

1. 辨证治疗

（1）邪热内结

慢性胃炎的中医特色疗法

Symptoms and signs: Fullness felt on the epigastric area, distension of the chest. Soft obdomem without pain, thrist and irritation, constipation, red tongue and slippery and rapid pulse.

Therapeutic methods: Clearing away heat, removing fullness and dispersing qi stagnation.

Recipes and herbs: Xiexin Tang. Ingredients: Dahuang, Huanglian and Huangqin. If the patient has distension of cheat and irritation, Gualou and Zhizi can be added to regulate qi and remove the fullness and distension of chest, to clear away heat and to remove any subsequent irritation in the chest. If the patient suffers from stomach reflux and vomiting, Zhuru and Xuanfuhua can be added to allow the stomach qi flow downwards naturally and to stop any further vomiting. If the patient suffers with extreme thirst, add Tianhuafen and Lianqiao to clear heat and increase body fluid. If the patient suffers with abdominal distension and constipation, add Mangxiao and Zhishi regulate movement of qi and soften the stool to relieve constipation.

(2) Accumulation of phlegm and dampness in the interior

Symptoms and sings: Fullness and distension of chest and abdomen, stomach reflux, a lot of thick phlegm, dizziness and vertigo, heaviness of the body and fatigue,

【证候】 心下痞满,胸膈满闷,按之濡软不痛,烦躁口渴,或见大便秘结,舌红,脉滑数。

【治法】 清热消痞,破结除满。

【方药】 泻心汤。药用大黄、黄连、黄芩。若胸闷心烦者,加瓜蒌、栀子以宽中行气,清热除烦;恶心呕吐者,加竹茹、旋覆花以降逆止呕;口渴欲饮者,加天花粉、连翘以清热生津;腹胀便秘者,加芒硝、枳实以软坚通便,行气消胀。

(2)痰湿内阻

【证候】 胸脘痞塞,满闷不舒,恶心欲吐,痰多或咯出不爽,头昏目眩,身重倦怠,舌质淡红、苔厚腻,脉

pale red tongue with thick greasy coating, slippery or wiry and slippery pulse.

Therapeutic methods: Eliminating dampness and resolving phlegm, regulating qi and removing fullness and distension of chest.

Recipes and herbs: Modified Pingwei San and Erchen Tang. Ingredients: Banxia, Fuling, Chenpi, Cangzhu, Houpo, Gancao and Shengjiang, etc. For patient with reverse flow of stomach qi and belching a lot, add Xuanfuhua and Daizheshi to resolve phlegm and descend stomach qi. If the patient has fullness and distension of chest, add Xiebai, Zhike and Gualou to regulate qi and remove fullness and distension of chest. If the patient has thick and yellow turbid phlegm together with thirst, dry mouth and irritation, add Huangqin and Huanglian to clear away heat-phlegm. For patient with exogenous evil symptoms, add Zisuye and Xiangfu to regulate and harmonise defensive qi.

(3) Liver qi stagnation

Symptoms and signs: Fullness and distension of chest and hypochondriac area, irritation, short tempered, yawning and sighing a lot, pale red tongue with thin white coating and wiry pulse.

Therapeutic methods: Soothing the liver to relieve depression, regulating qi to remove fullness with mass.

滑或弦滑。

【治法】 祛湿化痰,理气宽中。

【方药】 平胃散合二陈汤加减。
药用半夏、茯苓、陈皮、苍术、厚朴、甘
草、生姜等。若气逆不降,噫气不除
者,加旋覆花、代赭石以化痰降逆;胸
膈满闷较甚者,加薤白、枳壳、瓜蒌以
理气宽中;咯痰黄稠,心烦口干者,加
黄芩、黄连以清化痰热;兼有表证者,
加紫苏叶、香附以理气解表。

(3)肝郁气滞

【证候】 胸膈痞满,脘胁作胀,
心烦易怒,嗳气纳差,善太息,舌质淡
红、苔薄白,脉弦。

【治法】 疏肝解郁,理气除痞。

Recipes and herbs: Modified Sini San. Ingredients: Chaihu, Zhishi, Baishaoyao, Gancao, Cangzhu, Xiangfu, Chuanxiong, Shenqu and Shanzhizi, etc. If the patient has internal fire which is caused by qi stagnation and has bitter taste in mouth and irritation, add Longdancao and Chuanlianzi to clear away the liver fire. For patients with turbid fluid residing in the body and with thick and greasy tongue coating, add Fuling and Yiyiren to resolve the turbid fluid. If the patient has a lot of thick phlegm which causes stuffiness of chest, add Banxia and Chenpi to regulate movement of qi and resolve thick phlegm. If the patient's body constitution is weak and has weak zhong qi and at the same time same time suffers from liver qi stagnation, use formula "Simu Yinzi". However try not to use too many aromatic and dampness resolving herbs as these herbs often depletes qi. This formula containing Renshen, Binglang, Chenxiang and Wuyao not only regulate movement of qi and move qi stagnation but also strengthen zhenqi.

(4) Deficiency of the spleen and stomach

Symptoms and signs: Fullness and distension of chest and abdomen, variable abdominal distension feel hunger with no desire of eating, preference for heat and pressure, lethargy, diarrhea, pale pink tongue with thin white coating, deep and thin pulse or big, weak and empty pulse.

【方药】 四逆散加减。药用柴胡、枳实、白芍药、甘草、苍术、香附、川芎、神曲、山栀子等。若气郁化火，口苦心烦者，加龙胆草、川楝子以清肝泻火；湿浊内阻，舌苔厚腻者，加茯苓、薏苡仁以淡渗利湿；痰多胸闷，或咯痰不爽者，加半夏、陈皮以理气化痰；若素体虚弱，中气不足，而兼肝郁气滞者，不宜专用香燥耗气之剂，拟用四磨饮子为宜，方中用人参、槟榔、沉香、乌药以破滞降逆，兼益气扶正，使理气而不伤正，补气而不壅中。

(4) 脾胃虚弱

【证候】 心下痞满，胸膈不舒，腹胀时减、时宽、时急，饥而不食，喜热喜按，倦怠乏力，大便溏稀，舌质淡红、苔薄白，脉沉细或虚大无力。

Therapeutic methods: Tonifying qi, invigovating the spleen, ascending qingqi and descending dirty qi and morbid fluid.

Recipes and herbs: Modified Buzhong Yiqi Tang. Ingredients: Dangshen, Huangqi, Baizhu, Danggui, Shengma, Chaihu, Gancao, Zhike and Maiya, etc. For patients with spleen yang deficiency and intolerance of cold, add Fuzi and Wuzhuyu to warm the spleen channel and disperse cold. If the patient has a lot of dampness in the body and the tongue coating is thick and greasy and has poor appetite, add Fuling and Yiyiren to resolve dampness. For patients with abdominal distension and poor appetite, add Sharen and Shenqu to wake up the spleen via their aromatic properties and to resolve dirty morbid fluid and remove food stagnation. If the patient has qi stagnation with abdominal distension, add Muxiang and Foshou to regulate movement of qi and reduce abdominal distension. If the patient has liver qi stagnation, add Chuanlianzi and Yujin to sooth the liver and disperse stagnation of liver qi. If the patient suffers from deficiency of Mingmen fire with lower back pain and diarrhoea, add Rougui and Fuzi to warm up kidney Mingmen and strengthen the kidney and the spleen yang.

(5) Simultaneous occurence of cold and heat syndrome

【治法】 益气健脾,升清降浊。

【方药】 补中益气汤加味。药用党参、黄芪、白术、当归、升麻、柴胡、甘草、枳壳、麦芽等。若脾阳虚弱,畏寒怕冷者,加附子、吴茱萸以温经散寒;湿浊内盛,舌苔厚腻,脘闷纳呆者,加茯苓、薏苡仁以淡渗利湿;腹满纳差者,加砂仁、神曲芳香醒脾,化浊消食;气滞较甚,脘腹胀满者,加木香、佛手以理气除满;兼肝气郁滞者,加川楝子、郁金以疏肝化瘀;命门火衰,腰膝酸冷,大便溏稀者,加肉桂、附子以温补肾阳,脾肾同治。

(5) 寒热错杂

Symptoms and signs: Epigastric full distension, soft abdomen without pain with pressure, retching and nausea, thirst, dysphoria, dull pain in the epigasgtrium and abdomen, rumbling intestine, diarrhea, reddish tongue, whilte or yellow greasy fur, and deep wiry pulse.

Therapeutic methods: Treating the disease using herbs with cold and heat nature, harmonizing the middle jiao and relieve full distension.

Recipes and herbs: Modified Banxia Xiexin Decoction. Ingredients: Banxia, Huangqin, Ganjiang, Dangshen, Zhigancao, Huanglian and Dazao. In case of severe full distension in the epigastrium, Zhike and Houpo are added to relieve fullness by promoting qi-flow; in case of nausea and vomiting, Zhuru and Xuanfuhua are added to keep counterflow downstream and control vomiting; in case of severe spleen-yang insufficiency, middle-Jiao insufficiency-cold, chill and abdominal pain, Wuzhuyu and Fuzi are added to warm the channels and dispel cold; in case of diarrhea and severe dampness with thick greasy fur, Fuling and Cheqianzi are added to promote diuresis and control diarrhea; in case of epigastric oppression and poor appetite, Shenqu and Jiaoshanzhizi are added to promote digestion and remove food retension.

(6) Complex of insufficiency and excess syndromes

Symptoms and signs: Epigastric full distension, no

【证候】　心下痞满,按之柔软不痛,呕恶欲吐,口渴心烦,脘腹隐痛,肠鸣下利,舌质淡红、苔白或黄腻,脉沉弦。

【治法】　寒热并用,和中消痞。

【方药】　半夏泻心汤加减。药用半夏、黄芩、干姜、党参、炙甘草、黄连、大枣等。若脘痞腹胀较甚者,加枳壳、厚朴以行气除满;恶心呕吐者,加竹茹、旋覆花以降逆止呕;脾阳虚甚,中焦虚寒,畏寒腹痛者,加吴茱萸、附子以温经散寒;下利湿重,舌苔厚腻者,加茯苓、车前子以利湿止泻;脘闷纳差者,加神曲、焦山栀子以消食导滞。

(6) 虚实相兼
【证候】　心下痞满,按之不痛,

pain while pressed, retching and dysphoria, thirst with no desire for water, dry belching with malodor of food, rumbling intestine and diarrhea; reddish tongue, thickish white greasy fur or slimy greasy fur, and deep wiry pulse or weak large pulse.

Therapeutic methods: Harmonizing and supplementing the spleen-stomach, transforming rheum and clear away heat.

Recipes and herbs: Modified Shengjiang Xiexin Decoction. Ingredients: Shengjiang, Zhigancao, Dangshen, Ganjiang, Huanglian, Banxia, Dazao. In case of frequent belching with putrid sour breath, Maiya and Shenqu are added to promote digestion and remove food retention; in case of severe epigastric full distension, Zhike and Houpo are added to relieve distension by promoting qi-flow; in case of severe rumbling intestine and diarrhea, Fuling and Cheqianzi are added to reinforce the spleen, and control diarrhea.

2. Simple and proved formulae

(1) Caoguo

Ingredients: Proper amount of Caoguo.

Actions: Eliminating dampness and transforming turbidity.

Indications: Severe epigastric full distension due to internal obstruction of dampness turbidity.

呕恶心烦，口渴不欲饮，干噫食臭，肠鸣下利，舌质淡红、苔白腻偏厚或滑腻，脉沉弦或虚大无力。

【治法】 调补脾胃，化饮清热。

【方药】 生姜泻心汤加减。药用生姜、炙甘草、党参、干姜、黄连、半夏、大枣等。若嗳气频作，其味酸腐者，加麦芽、神曲以消食化积；脘腹痞满较甚者，加枳壳、厚朴以行气除满；肠鸣下利较甚者，加茯苓、车前子以健脾利水止泻。

2. 单方验方

（1）一味草果

【组成】 草果适量。

【功用】 祛湿化浊。

【适应证】 湿浊内阻引起的脘腹痞满。

Administration: Caoguo is roasted to show yellow and ground into powder; taken with warm water, 3 g each time, once or twice a day.

(2) Binglang Powder

Ingredients: Proper amount of Binglang.

Actions: Promoting digestion and removing food retension.

Indications: Severe epigastric full distension due to food retension.

Administration: Binglang burnt with nature preserved and ground into powder; taken with warm water, 5 g each time, once or twice a day.

(3) Dingxiang Caoguo Liangjiang Yin

Ingredients: Dingxiang, Caoguo and Gaoliangjiang, 3 g respectively, with a little brown sugar.

Actions: Warming the middle jiao and dispelling cold, eliminating dampness and relieving distension.

Indications: Epigastric full distension, relieved while warmed and pressed.

Administration: Dingxiang, Caoguo and Gaoliangjiang decocted with water, remove the dregs and obtain the fluids, with brown sugar for flavouring; take decoction, once or twice a day.

(4) Sharen Muxiang Hongtang Decoction

Ingredients: Sharen 3 g, Muxiang 3 g and Hongtang

【用法】 草果煨黄研细末,每次服 3 g,温开水送下,每日 1~2 次。

(2)槟榔散

【组成】 槟榔适量。

【功用】 消积导滞。

【适应证】 脘腹痞满有积滞者。

【用法】 槟榔烧存性,为末,每次服 5 g,温开水送下,每日 1~2 次。

(3)丁香草果良姜饮

【组成】 丁香、草果、高良姜各 3 g,红糖少许。

【功用】 温中散寒,化湿消痞。

【适应证】 脘腹痞满,喜热喜按。

【用法】 丁香、草果、高良姜水煎去渣取汁,加红糖调味,饮汤,每日 1~2 次。

(4)砂仁木香红糖饮

【组成】 砂仁 3 g,木香 3 g,红

6 g.

Actions: Regulating qi and harmonizing the stomach.

Indications: Spleen-stomach insufficiency, qi-stagnation and full distension.

Administration: Take the decoction made up of three herbs, once a day.

(5) Neijin Hujiao Powder

Ingredients: Jineijin 50 g and Hujiao 10 g.

Actions: Warming the middle jiao, reinforcing the stomach, promoting digestion and dissipate food retention.

Indications: Epigastric fullness and anorexia due to food retension and stomach-qi congestion.

Administration: Grind the two drugs into fine powder, take 6 g each time with warm boiled water.

(6) Biandou gruel

Ingredients: Baibiandou 250 g, Dangshen 12 g, and proper amount of rice.

Actions: Invigorating the spleen and supplementing the stomach.

Indications: Full distension due to spleen-stomach insufficiency.

Administration: Baibiandou is cooked first (its peel removed) and then Dangshen and rice are added and cooked into gruel, taken in the morning and evening.

糖 6 g。

【功用】 理气和胃。

【适应证】 脾胃虚弱,气滞痞满。

【用法】 以上三味水煎服,为 1 日剂量。

(5)内金胡椒散

【组成】 鸡内金 50 g,胡椒 10 g。

【功用】 温中健胃,消食化滞。

【适应证】 食积停滞,胃气壅塞引起的心下痞满、纳差者。

【用法】 上两味共为细末,每次服 6 g,温开水送下。

(6)扁豆粥

【组成】 白扁豆 250 g,党参 12 g,大米适量。

【功用】 健脾益胃。

【适应证】 脾胃虚弱所致的痞满。

【用法】 先煮白扁豆去其皮,再入党参、大米如常法煮粥。早晚服食。

(7) Radish Decoction

Ingredients: Proper amount of radish.

Actions: Rectifying qi and transforming phlegm, and dispelling full distension.

Indications: Full distension and discomfort due to internal stagnation of phlegm and qi.

Administration: Take radish soup.

3. External therapy

(1) Topical application of heated powder

Fupi 30 g and Shengjiangzha 15 g are mixed thoroughly and fried, and then enveloped in a piece of cloth, which is applied in the affected part. It is indicated in spleen-stomach insufficiency, middle-cold and severe full distension.

(2) 505 Shengong Yuanqi Bag (waist band) or Shoushi Jianshen Band is worn to cover the navel, for treating stomach-cold.

4. Acupuncture and moxibustion therapy

(1) Body needles

For the excess syndrome, the points of foot jueyin liver meridian and foot yangming stomach meridian are prescribed; filiform needles are used with draining method. The main points are Zusanli (ST 36), Tianshu (ST 25), Qihai (CV 6), Zhongwan (CV 12), Neiguan (PC 6), Qimen (LR 14), and Yanglingquan (GB 34). For the insufficiency

（7）白萝卜汤

【组成】 白萝卜适量。

【功用】 顺气化痰,消除痞满。

【适应证】 痰气内阻引起的胃脘痞满不舒。

【用法】 白萝卜煮汤饮服。

3. 外治法

（1）熨法

麸皮 30 g,生姜渣15 g,拌匀炒热后用布包裹,揉熨患处。适用于脾胃虚弱,中寒痞满。

（2）用 505 神功元气带或寿世健身带,系裹于脐部,主治胃寒痞满。

4. 针灸疗法

（1）体针

实证取足厥阴、足阳明经穴为主,以毫针刺,采用泻法,常取足三里、天枢、气海、中脘、内关、期门、阳陵泉等穴;虚证取背俞穴、任脉、足太阴、足阳明经穴为主,毫针刺,采用补法,常取脾俞、胃俞、中脘、内关、足三

syndrome, the points of Back-Shu, conception vessel and foot taiyin spleen meridian are prescribed, and filiform are used with supplementing method. The main points are Pishu (BL 20), Weishu (BL 21), Zhongwan (CV 12), Neiguan (PC 6), Zusanli (ST 36).

(2) Ear needle

The points of Spleen, Stomach, Sympathetic Nerve and Large Intestine are prescribed. For excess syndrome, the manupilation of acupunture is indicated and generally the penetrating depth is 2 - 3 fen, twisting with middle force clockwisely, and retained for 5 - 10 minutes, once daily. For the insufficiency syndrome, either embedding or manupilation of acupuncture is used. As a rule, the needles are embedded in 1 - 2 points by the same mothod as the above-mentioned. The needle is twisted with the small force counterclockwisely and embedded for 10 - 20 minutes, once every other day and 10 times a course.

5. Massage

(1) The patient is treated in the supine position and the points of Zhongwan (CV 12), Qihai (CV 6), Tianshu (ST 25), and Guanyuan (CV 4) are prescribed, being slowly pushed from Zhongwan (CV 12) to Qihai (CV 6) with Yizhichan, to-and-fro for 5 - 6 rounds, once daily, which is indicatded in the severe full distension belonging to excess syndrome.

里等穴。

（2）耳针

取脾、胃、交感、大肠。实证宜针刺法，一般刺入深度为2～3分，按顺时针方向中等幅度捻转，留针5～10分钟，每日1次。虚证宜采用埋针法，亦可用针刺法。埋针一般埋1～2个穴，采用针刺法时同上法，应按逆时针方向小幅度捻转，留针10～20分钟，隔日1次，10次为1个疗程。

5. 按摩

（1）患者取仰卧位，取中脘、气海、天枢、关元等穴，以一指禅法缓慢从中脘推至气海，往返5～6遍，每日1次，适用于痞满属实证者。

慢性胃炎的中医特色疗法

(2) The patient is treated in prone position and the points of Pishu (BL 20), Weishu (BL 21), Dachangshu (BL 25) and Changqiang (GV 1) are prescribed, pushed from top to bottom to and fro for 3 - 4 rounds till the feeling of heat fullness appears in local part, once a day, which is indicated in severe full distension belonging to the insufficiency syndrome.

(3) Self-massage: The patient himself rubs both his own palms till the palms feel hot, and then the palm centers are placed on subxiphoid area, kneading 30 rounds clockwisely and counterclockwisely respectively, twice or thrice daily, which is indicated in regulating qi-dynamics and dispersing severe full distension. Also with the right thumb, the point of right Zusanli (ST 36) is kneaded with gradually increased force, 50 rounds clockwisely and counterclockwisely respectively, till the patient feel sore, fullness, heaviness and numbness. Then by the same way, the left thumb is used to knead the left Zusanli, which is indicated in regulating qi activity and relieving severe full distension.

Section Three   Belching

It is clinically marked by the turbid qi countering up from the stomach through the esophagus into the mouth. It is often due to food retension, phlegm turbidity,

（2）患者取俯卧位，取脾俞、胃俞、大肠俞、长强等穴，用擦法，从上至下，往返 3～4 遍，至局部出现热胀感为宜，适用于痞满虚证。

（3）**自我按摩**：患者双手掌心相搓至热，然后用掌心置于剑突下，向顺时针和逆时针方向各揉 30 次，每日 2～3 次，能调理气机，消除痞满。也可以右手拇指按摩右足三里穴，力量逐渐加大，向顺时针和逆时针方向各揉 50 次，使局部有酸、胀、困、麻感为宜，然后以左手拇指以同样方法按摩左足三里穴，具有调理气机，减轻痞满之功。

（三）嗳气

嗳气指以胃中之浊气上逆，经食道由口排出为临床特征的病证。多因食滞、痰浊、痰热、气滞及脾胃亏虚

phlegm-heat, qi-stagnation and spleen-stomach insufficiency.

1. Treatment based on syndrome differentiation

(1) Food retension and non-digestion

Symptoms and signs: Eructating frequently after meal with putrid smell, anorexia, thick grimy fur and wiry slippery pulse.

Therapeutic methods: Promoting digestion and removing food retention, harmonizing the stomach to descend adverse flow of qi.

Recipes and herbs: Modified Baohe Pill. Ingredients: Shanzha, Shenqu, Maiya, fried Laifuzi, Chenpi, Banxia and Fuling. In case of constipation, Lianqiao is added to clear away heat; in case of severe full distension in chest and epigastrium, Zhishi and Houpo are added to move qi-flow and alleviate the middle.

(2) Phlegm turbidity obstructing the middle

Symptoms and signs: Eructation and oppression in the chest and epigastrium, severe nausea, dizziness in the early morning, slimy fur, and wiry slippery pulse.

Therapeutic methods: Dissipating phlegm and smoothing qi.

Recipes and herbs: Modified Erchen Decoction. Ingredients: Chenpi, Banxia, Fuling, Gancao, Sharen, Zhinanxing and Cangzhu. Without being cured for a long

所致。

1. 辨证治疗

（1）食滞不化

【证候】 食后嗳气频作，味腐而臭，厌食，苔厚浊，脉滑。

【治法】 消食导滞，和胃降逆。

【方药】 保和丸加减。药用山楂、神曲、麦芽、炒莱菔子、陈皮、半夏、茯苓。若大便秘结，苔黄腻者，加连翘以清热；胸脘痞满者，加枳实、厚朴以行气宽中。

（2）痰浊中阻

【证候】 嗳气、胸脘闷，恶心欲呕，晨起眩晕，苔腻，脉弦滑。

【治法】 化痰顺气。

【方药】 二陈汤加减。药用陈皮、半夏、茯苓、甘草、砂仁、制南星、苍术等。日久不愈，脾虚食少倦怠

time and having spleen-insufficiency, anorexia and fatigue, Dangshen and Baizhu are added to invigorate the spleen and supplement qi.

(3) Phlegm-heat accumulating in the interior

Symptoms and signs: Eructation, bitter taste in the mouth, oppression in the chest, distension in the epigastrium, yellow slimy fur and slippery rapid pulse.

Therapeutic methods: Clearing away heat and dissipating phlegm.

Recipes and herbs: Modified Wendan Decoction. Ingredients: Zhuru, Zhishi, Banxia, Chenpi, Fuling, Gancao and Jinyinhua. In case of yellow phlegm and cough, Xingren, and Beimu are added to transform phlegm and suppress cough.

(4) Spleen-stomach qi-insufficiency

Symptoms and signs: Paroxysmal eructation, belching with low voice, lassitude and weakness, poor intake of food,pale white fur and fine weak pulse.

Therapeutic methods: Invigorating the spleen and supplementing the stomach.

Recipes and herbs: Modified Xiangsha Liujunzi Decoction. Ingredients: Muxiang, Sharen, Fabanxia,Chenpi, Dangshen, Baizhu, Fuling, Gancao and Zhike. In case of obvious qi-counterflow and frequent eructation, Xuanfuhua and Daizheshi are added to keep counterflow

者,加党参、白术健脾益气。

（3）痰热内郁

【证候】 嗳气口苦,胸闷脘胀,苔黄腻,脉滑数。

【治法】 清热化痰。

【方药】 温胆汤加减。药用竹茹、枳实、半夏、陈皮、茯苓、甘草、金银花。伴痰黄咳嗽者,加杏仁、贝母化痰止咳。

（4）脾胃气虚

【证候】 嗳气时作时止,嗳声低弱,神疲乏力,食少,舌淡苔白,脉细弱。

【治法】 健脾益胃。

【方药】 香砂六君子汤加减。药用木香、砂仁、法半夏、陈皮、党参、白术、茯苓、甘草、枳壳等。若气逆明显,嗳气频作者,加旋覆花、代赭石以重镇降逆;四肢不温,泛吐清水者,加

downstream with heavy settling; in case of lacking warmth in the limbs and vomiting out much watery fluid, Paojiang and Wuzhuyu are added to warm the middle and dispel cold.

(5) Liver-qi invading the stomach

Symptoms and signs: Eructation and vomiting sour fluid, abdominal distension and hypochondrial pain, being more severe with mental depression, thin fur and wiry pulse.

Therapeutic methods: Soothing the liver and harmonizing the stomach.

Recipes and herbs: Modified Chaihu Shugan Decoction. Ingredients: Chaihu, Zhike, Baishaoyao, Gancao, Chenpi, Xiangfu, Yujin and Xuanfuhua. In case of frequent eructation, Chaihu is removed and Daizheshi is used instead to keep counterflow downstream with heavy settling; in case of bitter mouth and gastric upsetting, Chuanjianzi, Yanhusuo and Zhuru are added to clear away heat and to descend adverse flow of qi.

Section Four　Acid reflux

It refers to the acid reflux from the stomach which is then swallowed down, or to stomachache without acid reflux. It is also called "acid regurgitation" or "acid swallowing" which is mainly due to liver qi invading the stom-

炮姜、吴茱萸以温中散寒。

（5）肝气犯胃

【证候】 嗳气吐酸,腹胀胁痛,每因精神抑郁而加重,苔薄,脉弦。

【治法】 疏肝和胃。

【方药】 柴胡疏肝散加减。药用柴胡、枳壳、白芍药、甘草、青皮、陈皮、香附、郁金、旋覆花等。嗳气频作者,去柴胡,加代赭石以重镇降逆;口苦、嘈杂者,加川楝子、延胡索、竹茹以清热降逆。

（四）泛酸

泛酸是指酸水由胃中上泛,随即咽下,或只觉胃中酸酢而无酸水泛出。又称"吞酸"、"咽酸",多由肝气犯胃所致。

ach.

1. Treatment based on syndrome differentiation

(1) Heat syndrome

Symptoms and signs: Acid swallowing with dysphoria, dry throat, yellow fur, and wiry pulse.

Therapeutic methods: Purging the liver and clearing away fire.

Recipes and herbs: Zuojin Pill as main formula. Ingredients: Huanglian, Wuzhuyu, Wuzeigu and calcined Walengzi.

(2) Cold syndrome

Symptoms and signs: Acid swallowing with distension and oppression in the chest and epigastrium, eructation and putrid smell, white fur, and wiry moderate pulse.

Therapeutic methods: Warming and nourishing the stomach and the spleen.

Recipes and herbs: Modified Xiangsha Liujunzi Decoction. Ingredients : Muxiang, Sharen, Chenpi, Banxia, Dangshen, Baizhu, Fuling, Gancao and Wuzhuyu. In case of acid reflux after meal, less intake of food and thick fur, Shenqu and Guya are added to disperse stagnation and harmonize the stomach; in case of spleen disturbance due to damp turbidy, white slimy fur without being transformed, Sharen, Cangzhu, Huoxiang Peilan and the like to dissipate dampness

1. 辨证治疗

（1）热证

【证候】 吞酸而并见心烦,咽干,口苦,苔黄,脉多弦数。

【治法】 泄肝清火。

【方药】 左金丸为主方。药用黄连、吴茱萸、乌贼骨、煅瓦楞子等。

（2）寒证

【证候】 吞酸而并见胸脘胀闷,嗳气臭腐,苔白,脉多弦缓。

【治法】 温养脾胃。

【方药】 香砂六君子汤加减。药用木香、砂仁、陈皮、半夏、党参、白术、茯苓、甘草、吴茱萸等。若发于食后,纳少,苔厚,则加神曲、谷芽等以消滞和胃;如湿浊困脾,苔白腻不化者,可加砂仁、苍术、藿香、佩兰之类以化湿醒脾。

慢性胃炎的中医特色疗法

and arouse the spleen.

2. Simple and proved formulae

(1) Waleng Gancao Powder

Ingredients: Calcined Walengzi powder 150 g and Gancao powder 30 g.

Actions: Harmonizing the stomach and suppressing acid.

Indications: Hyperhydrochloria.

Administration: These two medicines are mixed thoroughly and contained in a bottle for use. Taking 6 g each time, swallowing with boiled mineral water, three times a day. After taking medicine, boiled water can also be drunk. The medicine can't be used without acid reflux.

(2) Jueming Muli Powder

Ingredients: Calcined Shijueming and calcined Muli with the same ratio.

Actions: Suppressing acid.

Indications: Hyperhydrochloria.

Administration: The two medicines are ground into a powder, taken 3 - 6 g each time, three times a day before meal.

(3) Muli Danke Powder

Ingredients: Calcined Muli and calcined egg shell with the same ratio.

Actions: Suppressing acid.

Indications: Hyperhydrochloria and gastric upset.

Administration: The two medicines are ground into a

2. 单方验方

（1）瓦楞甘草散

【组成】 煅瓦楞子末 150 g,甘草末 30 g。

【功用】 和胃制酸。

【适应证】 胃酸过多。

【用法】 上两味一起充分拌均匀后,再装入玻璃瓶内备用。每次服用 6 g,用矿泉水煮沸后吞服,每日 3 次,服后可随意饮用一些白开水。无泛酸者勿用。

（2）决明牡蛎散

【组成】 煅石决明、煅牡蛎各等份。

【功用】 制酸。

【适应证】 胃酸过多。

【用法】 共研细末,每次服 3～6 g,每日 3 次,饭前服。

（3）牡蛎蛋壳散

【组成】 煅牡蛎、煅鸡蛋壳等份。

【功用】 制酸。

【适应证】 胃酸过多,嘈杂。

【用法】 共研细末,每服 4.5 g,

慢性胃炎的中医特色疗法

powder, taken 4.5 g each time, three times daily.

(4) Gouwei Powder

Ingredients: One dog stomach, Baihujiao 5 g, glutinous rice 150 g and three pieces of ginger.

Actions: Warming the stomach, dissipating cold and suppressing acid.

Indications: Cold syndrome and acid swallowing.

Administration: Hujiao is ground and glutinous rice is steeped, both put into the dog stomach which is sewn with thread and steamed for two hours, taken one-thirds/fourths each time.

Section Five   Gastric upset

It refers to a feeling of hunger and emptiness with burning. Some could be relieved after meal and some patients could still have poor appetitie though upset in the stomach. Its common name is Caoxin or Xincao (heartburn). It is one of common symptoms of chronic gastritis and could be developed into epigastric pain and gastric reflux. There are different causes about it such as stomach heat, stomach insufficiency and blood insufficiency, which need different treatment according to different types.

1. Treatment based on syndrome differentiation

(1) Stomach heat

Symptoms and signs: Gastric upset with thirst, re-

每日 3 次。

（4）狗胃散

【组成】 狗胃 1 只,白胡椒 5 g,糯米 150 g,生姜 3 片。

【功用】 温胃散寒制酸。

【适应证】 寒证吞酸。

【用法】 先将胡椒研末,糯米浸湿,生姜纳狗胃内,外用针线缝好,蒸煮 2 小时后,分 3～4 次食下。

（五）嘈杂

嘈杂是指胃中有似饥饿、空虚伴灼热的一种感觉。或进食后可暂缓一时,或虽嘈杂而食欲并不佳。俗称"嘈心"或"心嘈"。嘈杂是慢性胃炎常见的一个症状,可发展为胃脘痛或反胃等。其病因有胃热、胃虚、血虚之不同,需分型施治。

1. 辨证治疗

（1）胃热

【证候】 嘈杂而兼见口渴喜冷,

lieved by coldness, foul breath and dysphoria, yellow fur and rapid pulse.

Therapeutic methods: Harmonizing the middle jiao and clearing away heat.

Recipes and herbs: Modified Wendan Decoction. Ingredients: Banxia, Chenpi, Gancao, Zhishi, Zhuru and Shengjiang. In case of excessive heat, Huanglian and Zhizi are added.

(2) Stomach insufficiency

Symptoms and signs: Gastric upset with tastelessness, epigastric distension after meals, pale tongue and vacuous pulse.

Therapeutic methods: Invigorating the spleen and harmonizing the stomach.

Recipes and herbs: Modified Sijunzi Decoction. Ingredients: Dangshen, Baizhu, Fuling, Huaishanyao, Biandou and Gancao.

(3) Blood insufficiency

Symptoms and signs: Gastric upset with sallow complexion, pale lips, palpitation, dizziness, reddish tongue and wiry pulse.

Therapeutic methods: Supplementing qi and nourishing blood.

Recipes and herbs: Modified Guipi Decoction. Ingredients: Huangqi, Dangshen, Baizhu, Fuling, Suanza-

口臭心烦,苔黄,或见脉数。

【治法】 和中清热。

【方药】 温胆汤加减。药用半夏、陈皮、甘草、枳实、竹茹、生姜等。热盛可加黄连、栀子之类。

（2）胃虚

【证候】 嘈杂而兼见口淡无味,食后脘胀,舌淡,脉虚。

【治法】 健脾和胃。

【方药】 四君子汤加减。药用党参、白术、茯苓、怀山药、扁豆、甘草等。

（3）血虚

【证候】 嘈杂而兼面色萎黄,唇淡,心悸头眩,舌淡红,脉细。

【治法】 益气养血。

【方药】 归脾汤加减。药用黄芪、党参、白术、茯神、酸枣仁、桂圆

oren, Guiyuanrou, Zhigancao, Danggui, Yuanzhi, Shengjiang and Dazao.

2. Chinese patent medicines

(1) Zuojin Pill

Ingredients: Huanglian and Wuzhuyu.

Actions: Clearing up liver-fire, harmonizing the stomach and relieving pain.

Indications: Gastric upset due to stomach heat.

Administration: Take 3－6 g each time, twice a day.

(2) Wuji Pill

Ingredients: Huanglian, Wuzhuyu and Baishaoyao.

Actions: Clearing away heat and harmonizing the stomach.

Indications: Gastric upset due to stomach heat.

Administration: Taking 6 g each time, twice a day.

(3) Guipi Pill

Ingredients: Renshen, Baizhu, Huangqi, Danggui, Fushen and Yuanzhi.

Actions: Supplementing qi, nourishing blood and invigorating the spleen.

Indications: Gastric upset with spleen and blood insufficiency.

Administration: Taking 6 g each time, twice a day.

(4) Liujunzi Pill

Ingredients: Dangshen, Chaobaizhu, Fuling, Mizhi-

肉、木香、炙甘草、当归、远志、生姜、大枣等。

2. 中成药

（1）左金丸

【组成】 黄连、吴茱萸。

【功用】 清肝泻火，和胃止痛。

【适应证】 胃热嘈杂。

【用法】 每次3～6g，每日2次。

（2）戊己丸

【组成】 黄连、吴茱萸、白芍药。

【功用】 清热和胃。

【适应证】 胃热嘈杂。

【用法】 每次6g，每日2次。

（3）归脾丸

【组成】 人参、白术、黄芪、当归、茯神、远志等。

【功用】 益气养血健脾。

【适应证】 脾虚血少嘈杂。

【用法】 每次6g，每日2次。

（4）六君子丸

【组成】 党参、炒白术、茯苓、蜜

gancao, Chenpi and Zhibanxia.

Actions: Supplementing qi, reinforcing the spleen, drying dampness and transforming phlegm.

Indications: Upset in the stomach and epigastrium.

Administration: Taking 6 g each time, twice a day.

Section Six   Vomiting

Vomiting is one of the main symptoms of chronic gastritis, due to failure of harmony and descending of qi, and ascending of counterflow qi.

1. Treatment based on syndrome differentiation

(1) Food retention

Symptoms and signs: Vomiting acid and putrid food, full distension in epigastrium and abdomen, eructation and anorexia, being aggravated after meal while alleviated after vomiting, foul or loose stool, or constipation, thick greasy fur and slimy replete pulse.

Therapeutic methods: Promoting digestion, eliminating stagnation, harmonizing the stomach to descend adverse flow of qi.

Recipes and herbs: Modified Baohe Pill. Ingredients: Shenqu, Shanzha, Laifuzi, Fuling, Chenpi, Banxia and Lianqiao. In case of fullness in the abdomen and constipation, Zhishi and Dahuang are added to flush the

炙甘草、陈皮、制半夏。

【功用】 益气健脾,燥湿化痰。

【适应证】 脾胃气虚引起的胃
脘嘈杂。

【用法】 每次 6 g,每日 2 次。

(六) 呕吐

呕吐是慢性胃炎一个主要症状,
是由于胃失和降,气逆于上引起的。

1. 辨证治疗

(1) 饮食停滞

【证候】 呕吐酸腐,脘腹胀满,
嗳气厌食,得食愈甚,吐后反快,大便
秽臭或溏薄或秘结,苔厚腻,脉滑实。

【治法】 消食化滞,和胃降逆。

【方药】 保和丸加减。药如神
曲、山楂、莱菔子、茯苓、陈皮、半夏、
连翘等。若腹满便秘者,加枳实、大
黄荡涤肠胃;胃寒者,去连翘,加干

stomach and intestine; in case of stomach cold, Lianqiao is removed and Ganjiang and Sharen are added instead; in case of stomach heat, Lugen is added.

(2) Internal obstruction of phlegm-rheum

Symptoms and signs: Vomiting watery fluid, phlegm and saliva, oppression in the epigastrium, anorexia, dizziness, papitation, white greasy fur and wiry pulse.

Therapeutic methods: Warming and transforming phlegm and rheum, harmonizing the stomach to descend adverse flow of qi.

Recipes and herbs: Modified Xiaobanxia Decoction and Lingguizhugan Decoction. Ingredients: Banxia, Shengjiang, Fuling, Guizhi, Baizhu and Ganchao. In case of internal obstruction by phlegm-rheum, and long-term depression turning into fire, Huanglian is added to clear away heat and transform phlegm.

(3) Liver-qi invading the stomach

Symptoms and signs: Vomiting and swallowing acid, frequent eructation, opression and pain in the chest and hypochodrial regions, red tongue margins, thin greasy fur, and wiry pulse.

Therapeutic methods: Soothing the liver, harmonizing the stomach, keeping counterflow downstream and suppressing vomiting.

Recipes and herbs: Modified Banxia Houpo Decoc-

姜、砂仁；胃热，加芦根。

（2）痰饮内阻

【证候】 呕吐多为清水痰涎，脘闷不食，头眩心悸，苔白腻，脉滑。

【治法】 温化痰饮，和胃降逆。

【方药】 小半夏汤合苓桂术甘汤加减。药如半夏、生姜、茯苓、桂枝、白术、甘草等。若痰饮内阻，郁久化热者，加用黄连以清热化痰。

（3）肝气犯胃

【证候】 呕吐吞酸，嗳气频繁，胸胁闷痛，舌边红、苔薄腻，脉弦。

【治法】 舒肝和胃，降逆止呕。

【方药】 半夏厚朴汤合左金丸

tion and Zuojin Decoction. Ingredients: Banxia, Houpo, Zisu, Banxia, Shengjiang, Fuling, Huanglian and Wuzhuyu. In case of liver depression turning into heat, Huanglian is added; in case of constipation, Dahuang ang Zhishi are added; in case of yin-impairment, Shashen and Maimendong are added.

(4) Spleen-stomach insufficiency cold

Symptoms and signs: Easy to vomit intermittently due to improper diet, lustreless complexion, fatigue, malaize, lack of strength, no desire to drink despite thirst, coldness in limbs, thin sloppy stool, pale tongue and soggy weak pulse.

Therapeutic methods: Warming the middle jiao, invigorating the spleen, harmonizing the stomach to descend adverse flow of qi.

Recipes and herbs: Modified Lizhong Decoction. Ingredients: Renshen, Baizhu, Ganjiang and Gancao. In case of severe stomach-cold and vomiting watery fluid, Paofuzi is added to increase the effects of warming the middle and dispelling cold.

(5) Stomach-yin insufficiency

Symptoms and signs: Frequent attacks of vomiting with intermittent retch, dry mouth and throat, no desire to eat despite hunger, red tongue with less liquid, and fine rapid pulse.

加减。药物如半夏、厚朴、紫苏、生姜、茯苓、黄连、吴茱萸等。若肝郁化热者,加黄连;便秘者,加大黄、枳实;化火伤阴者,加沙参、麦门冬。

（4）脾胃虚寒

【证候】 饮食稍有不慎,即易呕吐,时作时止,面色无华,倦怠乏力,口干而不欲饮,四肢不温,大便溏薄,舌质淡,脉濡弱。

【治法】 温中健脾,和胃降逆。

【方药】 理中丸加减。药如人参、白术、干姜、甘草等。胃寒较重,呕吐清水者,可加炮附子以增强温中散寒之功。

（5）胃阴不足

【证候】 呕吐反复发作,时作干呕,口燥咽干,似饥而不欲食,舌红少津,脉多细数。

Therapeutic methods: Supplementing and nourishing the stomach-yin, descending adverse flow of qi to suppress vomiting.

Recipes and herbs: Modified Maimendong Decoction. Ingredients: Taizishen, Maimendong, Jingmi, Gancao and Banxia. In case of severe qi-insufficiency and yin-impairment, Banxia may be removed and Xiyangshen are used instead of Taizishen and added with yin-nourishing medicines such as Shashen and Tianmengdong; in case of dry stool, Huomaren, Baimi and Gualuo are added; in case of severe vomiting, Zhuru and Pipaye are added.

2. Simple and proved formulae

(1) Xuanfu Daizhe Banxia Decoction

Ingredients: Xuanfuhua 10 g, Daizheshi 12 g, Banxia 12 g, Dangshen 12 g, Chuanlianzi 10 g, Chenpi 10 g, Dazao 6 g and Shengjiang 6 g.

Actions: Supplementing qi and reinforcing the stomach, descending adverse flow of qi to suppress vomiting.

Indications: Vomiting due to spleen-stomach insufficiency.

Adminstration: Decocted and taken, one dose a day.

(2) Dingxiang Jupi Decoction

Ingredients: Mudingxiang 3 and Chenpi 1 piece.

Actions: Descending adverse flow of qi to suppress vomiting.

【治法】 滋养胃阴,降逆止呕。

【方药】 麦门冬汤加减。药如太子参、麦门冬、粳米、甘草、半夏等。如气虚阴伤过甚者,可去半夏,改太子参为西洋参,并酌加养阴之品如沙参、天门冬等;大便干结者,加火麻仁、白蜜、瓜蒌等;呕吐较甚者,加竹茹、枇杷叶。

2. 单方验方

(1) 旋覆代赭半夏汤

【组成】 旋覆花 10 g,代赭石 12 g,半夏 10 g,党参 12 g,川楝子 10 g,陈皮 10 g,大枣 6 g,生姜 6 g。

【功用】 益气健胃,降逆止呕。

【适应证】 脾胃虚弱呕吐者。

【用法】 水煎服,每日 1 剂。

(2) 丁香橘皮饮

【组成】 母丁香 3 个,陈皮 1 块。

【功用】 降逆止呕。

Indications: Vomiting due to stomach-cold.

Administration: Taking hot decoction.

(3) Baihe Jizihuang Decoction

Ingredients: Baihe 45 g and Jizihuang 1.

Actions: Nourishing yin, reinforcing the stomach and clearing away heat.

Indications: Vomiting due to insufficiency of stomach-yin.

Administration: Baihe is washed and steeped for one night until the white foam appears, and the water is removed. Then the Baihe is decocted with clear water and boiled with Jizihuang. Taking the warm decoction, once or twice a day.

(4) Lugen Decoction

Ingredients: Fresh Lugen 90 g.

Actions: Clearing away heat, engendering body fluid and preventing vomiting.

Indications: Vomiting due to stomach-heat.

Administration: Taking the decoction.

(5) Jupi Gruel

Ingredients: Jupi 3 g, white rice 30 g and Shengjiang juice with moderate amount.

Actions: Harmonizing the stomach to suppress vomiting.

Indications: Various vomiting due to ascending coun-

【适应证】 胃冷呕吐。

【用法】 水煎热服。

（3）百合鸡子黄汤

【组成】 百合 45 g，鸡子黄 1 枚。

【功用】 养阴益胃清热。

【适应证】 胃阴不足的呕吐。

【用法】 用水洗百合浸一夜，当白沫出，去其水，再用清水煎，加鸡子黄，搅匀再稍煎沸即可。温服。每日 1～2 次。

（4）芦根饮

【组成】 新鲜芦根 90 g。

【功用】 清热生津止呕。

【适应证】 胃热呕吐。

【用法】 水煎服。

（5）橘皮粥

【组成】 橘皮 3 g，白米 30 g，生姜汁适量。

【功用】 和胃止呕。

【适应证】 胃气上逆的各种

terflow of stomach-qi.

Administration: Jupi and white rice cooked with water into gruel, taken with ginger juice.

3. External Therapy

Shengjiang and Banxia (one half each) are fried until heated, which is then wrapped in a piece of cloth and applied on epigastrical, navel and subumbilical areas. It is indicated in vomiting due to stomach-cold.

4. Acupuncture and moxibustion therapy

(1) Body acupuncture

The points on the Yangming meridian are mainly prescribed. Retaining the needle and moxibustions are for the cold syndrome while quickly withdrawing the needle without moxibustions are for heat syndrome. For liver-qi invading the stomach, reducing method is used in the foot jueyin liver-meridian points and supplementing method is used in the spleen meridian ponits; for middle-insufficiency syndrome, the supplementing the spleen is combined. Prescription: Neiguan (PC 6), Zhongwan (CV 12), Zusanli (ST 36), Gongsun (SP 4), Hegu (LI 4) and Jinjinyuye (Extra) are used for vomiting of heat syndrome; Shangwan (CV 13) and Weishu (BL 21) are used for vomiting of cold syndrome; Tanzhong (CV 17) and Fenglong (ST 40) are used for phlegm retension; Xiawan (CV 10) and Xuanji (CV 21) are used for food retension.

呕吐。

【用法】 橘皮与白米加水煎煮成粥,用姜汁冲服。

3. 外治法

生姜、半夏各等份,炒热,布包,熨胃脘、脐中及脐下等处。适宜于胃寒呕吐。

4. 针灸疗法

（1）体针

取阳明经穴为主。寒者留针多灸,热则疾出不灸。肝气犯胃,泻足厥阴经穴,补足阳明经穴;中虚宜兼补脾气。处方:内关、中脘、足三里、公孙。热吐用合谷、金津玉液;寒吐用上脘、胃俞;痰饮用膻中、丰隆;食积用下脘、璇玑;肝气犯胃用阳陵泉、太冲;中虚用脾俞、章门。

慢性胃炎的中医特色疗法

(2) Ear acupnctuture

The points of Wei, Liver, Sympathetic, Subcortical, Shenmen points are prescribed. Two or three points are selected for each treatment, with a strong stimulation and retaining the needle for 20 – 30 minutes, once daily or every other day, which is mainly for pain in the epigstrium and stomach.

5. Massage

(1) Method of finger pressing Neiguan (PC 6)

The point of Neiguan (PC 6) in one side is pressed by himself with the middle finger of the other hand, or by other person's finger until having feeling of distensional pain, lasting for about one minute.

(2) Method of pressing Zhituxue

The points of Zhituxue are on the palm surface, straight below the wrist across the middle striation. The point is point-pressing for 2 – 3 minutes; pressing one side for mild vomiting and pressing both sides for the severe.

In addition, the methods for vomiting of cold syndrome are to tonify Pijing and warm Weijing, push Banmen from Hengwen, knead Wailaogong, push Sanguan and Tianzhugu, and knead Zhongwan; the methods for vomiting of heat syndrome are to clear Piwei and Dachang, reduce Liufu, move Neibaguan, push Banmen from Hengwen, and push Tianzhugu and Xiaqijiegu.

（2）耳针

选用胃、肝、交感、皮质下、神门等穴，每次取 2～3 穴，强刺激，留针20～30 分钟，每日或隔日 1 次。用于气滞血瘀引起的胃脘痛。

5. 按摩

（1）指压内关穴法

可自己用一手中指按压另一手内关穴，也可由他人按压，按压至有胀痛感，并持续 1 分钟左右。

（2）按止吐穴

止吐穴在手掌面，腕横纹正直下0.5 处。点按穴位 2～3 分钟，呕吐轻者点按一侧，重者点按双手。

此外，寒证呕吐，补脾经、温胃经，横纹推向板门、揉外劳宫、推三关、推天柱骨、揉中脘。热证呕吐，清脾胃、清大肠、退六腑、运内八卦、横纹推向板门、推天柱骨、推下七节骨。

慢性胃炎的中医特色疗法

Chapter Four   Self-Care for Chronic Gastritis

Section One   Emotional adjustment

Of the multiple factors related to chronic gastritis, the emotional factors play an important role. Particularly, the patients with chronic atrophic gastritis who would consider it as an possible precancerous change often manifest various degrees of anxiety and fear, being extremely worried all day long, depressed, agitated, or even disheartened leading to insomnia. This manifestation is no good for the health which in turn affects the treatment and even increases the severity of the disease. Therefore it is the key for the patients to adjust the mind and have more confidence to overcome the disease. Generally the patients with the disease should adjust his own emotion, keeping in a good mood as to increase therapeutic effect, through communicating with the family members, colleagues and friends and joining some leisure acitivities such as listening to the cheerful light music and social dance.

Section Two   Dieting

Chronic gastritis is also concerned with unhealthy

四、慢性胃炎的摄生调护

（一）调节情志

慢性胃炎的发病因素较多，其中情志因素起着重要的作用，尤其是慢性萎缩性胃炎患者因为该病有癌变的可能，都存在不同程度的焦虑和恐惧，整日忧心忡忡，精神抑郁，或烦躁易怒，或悲观失望，造成失眠、多虑等。而上述表现不仅对身体无益，还影响治疗，甚至加重病情。因此，慢性胃炎患者康复的关键在于调养精神，树立战胜疾病的信心。平时要保持愉快的心情，多与家庭成员、同事、朋友相互交流，还可根据各人的爱好参加一些轻松愉快的文娱活动，如听听欢快流畅的乐曲，跳跳交谊舞等，以调节自己的情志，有益于疾病的治疗与康复。

（二）节制饮食

慢性胃炎与不良的饮食习惯也

diet habits such as liking spicy food as well as drinking and smoking, which should be given up. Moreover the good diet habits should be established, including samll frequent meals, swallowing slowly and thoroughly, moderating food intake, avoiding colder, hotter, harder and stickier food, in order to relieve gastric retension, protect gastric mucosa and then prevent the progress, causing better theraputic result.

Section Three　Treating related diseases

The related diseases such as stomachtitis, cholecystitis and bile regurgitation should be cured.

Besides, the patients should avoid the drugs having strong irritation to gastric mucosa, especially the antipyretic and analgesic such as aspirin, anticipate moderate exercise to enhance immunity which is beneficial to the early recovery, and pay more attention to food hygeine and prevent infection of HP.

有一定的关系,所以首先应注意戒除不良的饮食嗜好,如不吃辛辣刺激性食物,戒掉烟酒等。再则要养成良好的饮食习惯,饮食宜少吃多餐,细嚼慢咽,不要过饥过饱,避免过冷、过热及过硬、过黏的食物,以减轻胃的负担,保护胃黏膜,从而有效地防止本病的进一步发展,有利于治疗。

(三) 治疗相关疾病

如患有口腔炎、胆囊炎、胆汁反流等疾病者,应积极治疗,消除原发病。

此外,应避免服用对胃黏膜刺激性较强的药物,特别是解热镇痛药如阿司匹林等;可进行适当的体育活动及锻炼,增强机体的免疫力,以利于身体的早日康复;注意饮食卫生,防止幽门螺杆菌感染,从而减少本病的发生。

慢性胃炎的中医特色疗法

Part Three   Experience of Famous Senior TCM Doctors

Chapter One   Experience from Professor Deng Tietao

Section One   View on etiology and pathogenesis

Professor Deng thinks that the diseases are due to dysphoria, stress and over-thinking which may insidiously damage yang-qi and yin-humour; it is due to long term of improper diet and loss of regimen which damage the later heaven; it is also due to insufficiency of the earlier heaven, loss of later heaven and gross disorder. In the view of syndrome differentiation of TCM, the essential mechenism of the diseases is insufficiency in root and excess in tip. The insufficiency is mainly manifested as insufficiency of spleen-stomach, the spleen being Yang-qi insufficiency and the stomach being yin-humour insuficiency, which are the premise and nature of the pathogenesis. The excess of the diseases is mainly secondary to the insufficiency impairment. For examples, the spleen-qi

下篇 名老中医治验

一、邓铁涛教授治验

（一）对病因病机的认识

邓教授认为本病多由烦劳紧张，思虑过度，暗耗阳气，损伤阴液而引起；亦可因长期饮食失节，失于调养，致使后天损伤而发病；还可因先天不足，后天失养，大病失调所致。从中医学辨证角度来看，本病基本的病理机制为本虚标实。其虚，主要为脾胃亏虚，脾亏虚于阳气，胃亏虚于阴液，此为病发的前提和本质。本病之实，多为虚损之后所继发，如脾气亏虚，无力推动血液运行，血滞成瘀阻络，此为一；脾失健运，湿浊不化，痰湿停聚，此为二；瘀阻湿郁，加之阴液亏损，则易引致虚火妄动，此为三。脾

insufficiency isn't capable of promoting blood resulting in blood stasis and channel blockage; secondly, spleen failure to transport, dampness turbidity falilure to be transformed and the phlegm-dampness stasis and accumulation; thirdly, blood stasis and damp retension with yin-humour insufficiency tend to result in stirring-up of insufficiency-fire. Because of the spleen-yang insufficiency, there appear malaise, distension and oppression in the abdomen and epigastrium, anorexia, pale complexion, enlarged pale tongue with teeth marks and weak pulse; because of stomach-yin insufficiency, there appear dull pain and even heartburn in the stomach, flaccid tongue, less or no fur, rapid thready pulse; because of blood stasis obstructing channel, there appear severe pain in the gastrium and abdomen, severe tenderness in the upper abdomen and lumbar back, dark tongue and lip, petechia and ecchymosis on the tongue sides; because of retension of phlegm-damp, there appear distension and oppression in the epigastrium and abdomen, nausea, eructation, and even vomiting; because of internal heat from yin-insufficiency, there appear low fever, feverish sensation in the five centers, irritable mood, heartburn and dry stool.

阳亏虚,故见身倦乏力,脘腹胀闷,纳呆,体重下降,面色淡白,舌胖淡嫩,齿印,脉虚弱;胃阴亏损,则见胃部隐痛,甚则烧灼痛,舌嫩苔少或光剥,脉细数;血瘀阻络,则胃脘疼痛明显,上腹及背部夹脊压痛明显,舌暗、唇暗,舌边见瘀点、瘀斑;痰湿凝聚,则脘腹胀闷,恶心,嗳气,甚至呕吐;阴虚内热则见低热,五心烦热,急躁易怒,烧灼感,大便干燥等。

Section Two   Therapeutic experience and characteristics

The principle of treatment in this disease is to supplement the spleen-qi and nourish the stomach-yin, which is emphasized as the basis of the treatment. However, it is difficult to strengthen the efficacy of principle therapy without removing excess exterior syndrome and therefore promoting circulation, removing stasis, eliminating dampness, dissipating phlegm and clearing away insufficiency heat are important measures that couldn't be overlooked. The essential formula is Taizishen 30 g, Yunfuling 2 g, Huaishanyao 12 g, Shihu 12 g, Huancao 9 g, Maiya 30 g, Gancao 5 g, Danshen 12 g and Biejia 30 g (decocted prior to other drugs). In this formula, Taizishen, Yunfuling, Huaishanyao, Maiya and Gancao are used to supplement the spleen-stomach and tonify qi; Shihu, Huancao and Huaishanyao are used to rescue the damaged stomach-yin; Danshen and Biejia are used to reinforce yin and activate collaterals, free vessels and dispel stasis, with clearing away insufficiency-heat. In case of severe qi-insufficiency of the spleen-stomach, Huangqi and Baizhu are added or Shenxu is stewed separately; in case of severe dampness turbidity, Biandou and Yiyiren are added; in case of stagnation of liver-qi, Suxinhua,

（二）治疗经验与特色

对于本病的治疗，邓教授制订了补脾气、养胃阴的治疗大法，并强调此法是治疗的根本。但标实不除，则不能很好地固本，所以活络祛瘀，除湿化痰，清退虚热，也是不可忽略的重要措施。基本方为：太子参 30 g，云茯苓 12 g，怀山药 12 g，石斛 12 g，环草 9 g，麦芽 30 g，甘草 5 g，丹参 12 g，鳖甲 30 g（先煎）。方中用太子参、云茯苓、怀山药、麦芽、甘草以培补脾胃健运其气；用石斛、环草、怀山药急救已伤之胃阴，用丹参、鳖甲益阴活络，通脉祛瘀兼清虚热。脾胃气虚较甚者加黄芪、白术或参须另炖；湿浊偏重者加扁豆、薏苡仁等；肝气郁结者加素馨花、合欢皮、郁金等；疼痛明显者加木香、延胡索、佛手等；嗳气频作者加代赭石、旋覆花等；大便干结者加火麻仁、郁李仁等。

慢性胃炎的中医特色疗法

Hehuanpi and Yujin are added; in case of severe pain, Muxiang, Yanhusuo and Foshou are added; in case of frequent eructation, Daizheshi and Xuanfuhua are added; in case of dry stool, Huomaoren and Yuliren are added.

Chronic gastritis mostly occurs due to acquired factors, which may result in root weakness with damaged digestive function of spleen-stomach. Therefore the method in eagerness to obtain quick effect using some rich herbs to warm and supplment excessively should be avoided. Otherwise, the stomach-qi would be stagnated and the stomach-yin would be burnd up. Meanwhile, some greasy tonics aren't suitable for protecting the stomach-yin emergently which could prevent the recovery of stagnated yang-qi of the spleen. Besides for the same reason, excessively activating channel and removing blood-stasis would break blood too much and excessively clear away insufficiency-heat would damage yang too much. Professor Deng thinks that, in order to treat the disease and reinforce the original qi, it is preferable to use Taizishen, Huaishanyao, Yunfuling and Zhigancao. Though their supplementing effect are less than Dangshen and Huangqi, these four drugs wouldn't stagnate qi and encourage the evil fire. Paradoxically, Maiya is used to promote intake of food, which is appropriate for the patient with

慢性胃炎是伤于后天,其本既虚,脾胃消化吸收功能甚差,故培补不能急功求成,骤投大温大补之厚剂。如按此法,只能滞其胃气,灼其胃阴。同时,救护胃阴亦不宜用过于滋腻之品,以免壅阻脾脏阳气的恢复。此外,活络祛瘀要防破血太过,清退虚热要防伤阳,亦同上理。认为治疗本病培元时,宜用太子参、怀山药、云茯苓、炙甘草等,虽补气之力不及党参、黄芪,但不会滞气助火;再反佐以麦芽使之易于受纳,这对于消化吸收功能甚差、胃阴已伤的患者,是恰如其分的。至于救胃阴,石斛、环草、怀山药最为适宜;活络通瘀、清降虚热,丹参配鳖甲较为妥贴;至于化湿浊,宜选用扁豆、云茯苓等药性较平和的药物,切忌用温燥之品,因为易伤元气与胃阴,犯虚虚之弊。

decreased digestive function and damaged stomach-yin. For rescuing the stomach-yin, Shihu, Huancao and Huaishanyao are the best candidates; for activating channel and removing stasis, Danshen combined with Biejia are more suitable; for dissipating damp turbidity, some medicines with moderate nature such as Biandou and Yunfuling are chosen and the medicine with warm and dry nature shouldn't be used which tend to damage the original qi and stomach-yin and therefore yield the mistake called as "weaken the weakness".

This chronic disease has such a long course that it may finally affect kidney. In terms of Five Elements theory, spleen and stomach correspond to earth and liver to wood; the liver-qi tends to invade the spleen-qi by taking the advantage of spleen-insufficiency; so the relationship between the liver and the kidney as well as the lung and the spleen shouldn't be neglected, and in order to solve the problem in the principle aspect, the medicines to nourish the lung, the liver and the kidney could be choosed at appropriate timing. Meanwhile some predisposing factors should be avoided by giving up smoking and drinking, treating the chronic foci in the mouth and throat, and avoiding overfatigue and nervousness. Good dietary habits should be emphasized and it is beneficial to avoid irritant, too hot or too cold, and tough food, and

本病乃慢性疾病,病程较长,日久穷必及肾。脾胃属土,肝属木,脾虚往往使肝气乘之,故治疗时不能忽视与肝肾的关系,同时亦应注意肺脾的关系,故应抓主要矛盾,于适当之时选加调养肺、肝、肾之品。同时,注意消除可能致病的因素,如戒除烟酒,治疗口腔、咽喉部慢性病灶,忌用对胃有刺激的药物,避免过劳及精神紧张。注意饮食,戒刺激性、过热、过冷及粗糙食物,以软食为宜,少食多餐,细嚼慢咽。

to take soft food, small and frequent meals, by slowly chewing and swollowing.

Section Three   Report of typical cases

Ms Wu, 47 years old, the date of first visit: Mar. 9, 1978.

History: The patient has the stomach disease for over 30 years. In recent three months, the illness had been worse, presenting anorexia, loss of weight and intermittent vomiting. The diagnostic gastrofiberoscopy: superficial atrophic gastritis and duodenal bulbar inflammation, gastroptosis. There was no relief after treatment. After admission to this hospital, vomiting was suppressed through treatment with fluid infusion, antispasmoidic, analgesic, sedative and anti-inflammation agents. Continued treatment with digestives, the patient became better and could eat semifluid food. However, because of less daily intake of about 50 grams, the patient's weight continued to reduce and weight loss in total was as much as 12 kilograms in past months.

Examination: The findings are sallow complexion with less luster, dark lip, dark and tender tongue with tooth-mark, stasis specles and macules at the tip and around tongue sides, nearly complete peeling fur, only sparce curdy fur at the root; wiry fine pulse in the left

（三）验案介绍

吴某，女，47 岁。初诊：1978 年 3 月 9 日。

【病史】　患胃病 30 余年，近 3 个月来加剧。纳呆消瘦，间歇性呕吐，某医院作纤维胃镜检查诊断：浅表性萎缩性胃炎及十二指肠球炎、胃下垂。经治疗未见好转。入本院后经补液、解痉止痛、镇静、消炎等治疗，呕吐止，继以助消化药后渐好转，能进半流质食物，但每日进食只 50 g 左右，故体重仍在下降，几个月来共减重12 kg。于 3 月 9 日来诊。

【诊查】　诊见面色黄滞少华，唇黯，舌黯嫩、齿印、舌边尖有瘀点瘀斑，苔剥近于光苔，只于舌根部尚有疏落之腐苔，脉左弦细，右虚寸弱尺更弱。低热，大便 7 天未行，背部夹

handwhile feeble pulse in the right hand, weak inch pulse and weaker cubit pulse. Slight fever, constipation for seven days and multiple tender points in the lumbar back.

Syndrome differentiation: The disease is due to extremely insufficiency of qi and yin, loss of warmth and nourishment, failure to promote circulation and static blood obstructing vessels and channels.

Therapeutic methods: Supplementing qi, reinforcing the spleen and harmonizing the stomach, and to nourishing yin and rescuing the fluid, combined with activating blood and freeing the vessels as well as clearing the insufficient heat.

Formula: Taizishen 24 g, Yunfuling 12 g, Huaishanyao 12 g, Shihu 9 g, Huancao 9 g, Danshen 12 g, Biejia 30 g (decocted first), Maiya 18 g and Gancao 5 g.

Addition: Shenxu 9 g, stewed, once a week for seven times.

The second visit: On March 15, low fever disappeared and patient felt better in motional status with slightly improved appetite but constipation still existed; the comoplexion was truning lustrous gradually, dark lips, tender dark tongue and thin white fur at the middle and the root tongue. The treatment was continued with the first principle, added with Baizhu 9 g and Huomaren

脊有多处压痛点。

【辨证】 此乃气阴大虚,胃失煦养,血失鼓动,瘀阻脉络之候。

【治法】 宜补气健脾和胃,养阴救津,佐以活血通络,兼退虚热。

【处方】 太子参 24 g,云茯苓 12 g,怀山药 12 g,石斛 9 g,环草 9 g,丹参 12 g,鳖甲 30 g(先煎),麦芽 18 g,甘草 5 g。7 剂。

另:参须 9 g,每周炖服 1 次。

二诊:3 月 15 日,低热退,精神较好,食量稍增,唯大便尚秘结难排,面色由黄滞转稍有润泽,唇黯,舌嫩色黯,苔薄白(中根部)。治守前法,于前方中加白术 9 g、火麻仁 18 g。另炖服参须 9 g,每 5 天 1 次。

18 g; Shenxu 9 g was stewed and taken every 5 days.

The third visit: On March 22, low fever appeared again with feeling of hunger while constipation was relieved by Kaisailu. The tender tongue was enlarged and dark with ecchymosis on sides, with thin white moist fur and slow thin weak pulse (slight wiry in the right).

Formula: Taizishen 30 g, Yunfuling 12 g, Huaishanyao 18 g, Shihu 1 g, Huancao 9 g, Danshen 15 g, Biejia 30 g (decocted first), Maiya 18 g, Baihe 15 g and Gancao 4.5 g, for 7 doses. Stewed Shenxu 9 g was taken every 4 days.

The fourth visit: On March 29, the patient complained of headache and dizziness. The menstruation came 3 days ago and would be clear the next day. She had better appetite and ate 25 g rice for each meal, having dark pale lips, dark tender tongue with less ecchymosis, thin white fur (specially thin at tip), and thready rapid pulse (slightly wiry in the right). Then the former formula was added with Baihe (changed to be 24 g), Zhigancao 6 g while Danshen was removed. The patient was ordered to take modified formula added with Danshen 18 g and Baihe 30 g for totally 10 doses and stewed Shenxu 9 g was taken every 4 dyas.

The fifth visit: On April 12, the patient gained

三诊:3月22日。又见低热,开始有饥饿感,大便仍靠开塞露始能排出。舌嫩胖色黯,舌边有瘀斑,苔薄白润,脉缓细弱,右稍弦。

【处方】 太子参30 g,云茯苓12 g,怀山药18 g,石斛9 g,环草9 g,丹参15 g,鳖甲30 g(先煎),麦芽18 g,百合15 g,甘草4.5 g。7剂。

另炖参须9 g,每4天1次。

四诊:3月29日。头痛头晕,月经来潮已3天,翌日将净,胃纳转佳,每餐能进25 g米饭,唇黯稍淡,舌黯嫩,瘀斑稍减少,苔薄白,尖部少苔,脉细数,右稍弦。照上方加百合24 g、炙甘草6 g,去丹参(因月事未完)。并嘱从第4天起加丹参18 g,百合加至30 g,连服10剂。仍4天炖服参须9 g1次。

五诊:4月12日。体重比入院

weight of 3 kg compared with the lowest weight at admission(41 kg), with feeling of hunger, better complexion and plumpy face. The dark tongue with recurrent white fur and less ecchymosis over the sides and slight weak pulse were observed.

Formula: Taizishen 30 g, Yunling 12 g, Huaishanyao 18 g, Huancao 18 g, Guiban 30 g (decocted first), Baihe 30 g, Suxinhua 6 g, Maiya 30 g, Danshen 18 g, Daozao 4 and Zhigancao 6 g, for 7 doses.

The sixth visit: On April 18, the condition was improved. The gastrofiberscopy on April 15 revealed chronic superficial gastritis (not atrophic gastritis as before). Biopsy showed chronic inflammatory cells. The dark pale tongue, thin white fur over whole tongue, smaller ecchymosis and slow but slight wiry pulse were observed.

Formula: The former formula was modified with Huancao 15 g, Baihe 24 g and Danshen 15 g added, for 15-day administration.

The seventh visit: On May 3, the patient felt better and ate 150 - 200 g rice each day with moist complexion though dark in cheeks. The pale lip, tender pale tongue with shallow ecchymosis, thin white fur, and thready pulse in the left and wiry pulse in the right were observed.

后最低时(41 kg)增加 3 kg 多,有饥饿感,面色转好,面部较前饱满。舌黯,白苔复长,舌边瘀斑减少,脉强稍弱。

【处方】　太子参 30 g,云茯苓 12 g,怀山药 18 g,环草 18 g,龟版 30 g(先煎),百合 30 g,素馨花 6 g,麦芽 30 g,丹参 18 g,大枣 4 枚,炙甘草 6 g。7 剂。

六诊:4 月 18 日。病况继续好转,4 月 15 日作纤维胃镜检查:慢性浅表性胃炎(已非萎缩性胃炎)。活检亦为慢性炎症细胞。舌质淡黯、苔薄白(全舌有苔),舌边瘀斑缩小,脉缓稍弦。

【处方】　照上方环草改为 15 g,百合 24 g,丹参 15 g。共服半个月。

七诊:5 月 3 日。患者自觉良好,每天可食 150～200 g 米饭,面色转润,颧部仍黯。唇淡,舌质淡嫩,有瘀斑,但色变浅,苔薄白,脉左细右弦。

Formula: Taizishen 30 g, Huangqi 15 g, Yunfuling 12 g, Baizhu 9 g, Huaishanyao 18 g, Guiban 30 g (cooked first), Huancao 19 g, Danshen 15 g, Maiya 30 g, Dazao 4 and Gancao 5 g.

The patient continually took the medicines after discharge and rested for half a year before returning to work. No recurrence was noticed during 7 years of follow-up.

Chapter Two   Experience from Professor Zhang Zesheng

Section One   Clinical experience and characteristics

Atrophic gatritis is chracterized by full distension and pain in epigastrium and abdomen, relieved by pressing and kneading or after eating. It is usually accompanied with belching, pale tongue with white fur and deep pulse. Most of the cases could be differentiated as middle-insufficiency with stomach-cold or qi stagnation. The treatment is to warm the middle and reinforce digestion. So Guishaoliujun and Xiaojianzhong (Decoction)modified are commonly applied. In these formula, dose of Baishaoyao is larger than that of Guizhi to warm the mid-

【处方】 太子参 30 g,黄芪 15 g,云茯苓 12 g,白术 9 g,怀山药 18 g,龟版式 30 g(先煎),环草 12 g,丹参 15 g,麦芽 30 g,大枣 4 枚,甘草 5 g。

患者带药出院,继续到杭州疗养半年后恢复工作。追踪观察 7 年余,未见反复。

二、张泽生教授治验

(一)治疗经验与特色

萎缩性胃炎临床主要表现为脘腹胀满疼痛,喜揉喜按,得食稍缓,伴有嗳气,舌淡苔白,脉沉等。本病以中虚气滞或中虚胃寒证居多,治宜温中健运为主,常用归芍六君和小建中汤加减,方中白芍药用量重于桂枝,旨在温中缓急。但虚则气滞,病久入络,往往又挟有气滞血瘀,可参入枳壳、紫苏梗、佛手片、木香、红花、当归等,以行气滞,化瘀血。

dle and relieve spasmoidic pain. Since insufficiency could result in qi-stagnation and disease for long-term could enter channels, such medicines as Zhike, Zisugeng, Foshoupian, Muxiang, Honghua and Danggui are used to free qi stagnation and resolve blood stasis.

Section Two   Report of typical cases

1. Mr. Luo, male, 50, date of the first visit: March 6, 1976.

He had suffered form right epigastric pain for 5 – 6 years that aggravated in the last 2 years. The pain was even continuous everyday and even so severe as to sweat, relieved by heating or pressing. The diagnostic gastroscopy by Drum-building Hospital revealed chronic atrophic gastritis and diverticula in middle piece of esophagus. The pathologic report showed moderate atrophic gastritis, mild chronic inflammation in mucosa of duodenal bulb, fundus and lesser curvature. The purple lips, pale tongue, white fur and deep wiry were observed. The syndrome differentiation was middle-insufficiency and qi-stagnation, and treatment principle is to adjust the middle and harmonize stomach.

Formula: Dangshen 15 g, Chaodanggui 9 g, Chuanguizhi 3 g, Hangbaishaoyao 9 g, Banxia 9 g, Guangmuxiang 5 g, Guangchenpi 6 g and Zhigancao 3 g.

（二）验案介绍

1.罗某,男,50岁。初诊:1976年3月6日。

右上腹疼痛五六年,最近两年来病情加重,甚则每天持续疼痛不止,痛甚出汗,喜热喜按,经鼓楼医院胃镜检查为慢性萎缩性胃炎、食管中段憩室。病理报告为中度萎缩性胃炎,十二指肠球部、胃底小弯黏膜组织示轻度慢性炎症。脉沉弦,舌淡苔白,唇紫。中虚气滞,拟调中和胃治之。

【处方】 党参15 g,炒当归9 g,川桂枝3 g,杭白芍药9 g,半夏9 g,广木香5 g,广陈皮6 g,炙甘草3 g。

The second visit: On Jan. 19, 1977, the patient said that stomachache was relieved obviously after continuous administration of this formula for over 200 doses. The gastroscopy check-up by Drum-building Hospital revealed chronic atrophic gastritis. The pathologic report showed mild atrophic gastritis in mucosa of antrum, lesser curvature and posterior wall of the gastric corpus.

Formula: Banxia and Muxiang were removed while Honghua 9 g and Wumeitan 5 g are added instead.

The third visit: On June 13, a letter from the patient said that after taking 150 doses of this formula, no stomachache attacked and the conditions were stable except perspiration.

Formula: Shengjiang 2 slices and Dazao 4 were added to regulate ying and wei to consolidate remission.

On December 30, the patient came to Nanjing for check-up. The stomachache had disappeared and normal diet and excretion, with increased weight gain. The gastroscopy by Drum-building Hospital on Febuary 1, 1978 revealed subsiding of atrophic gastritis. The pathologic study showed mild atrophic gastritis in lesser curvatrure of the fundus and severe superficial gastritis of gastric body. The patient was then ordered to take the medicine

1977年1月19日二诊：上方连服200余剂，胃痛明显减轻。在鼓楼医院复查胃镜印象：慢性萎缩性胃炎。病理报告：胃窦大弯、胃体后壁黏膜组织、胃体小弯为轻度萎缩性胃炎。

上方去半夏、木香，加红花9 g、乌梅炭5 g。

6月13日三诊：患者来信云，上方又服150剂，胃痛未作，证情稳定，惟出汗较多。

原方加生姜2片、大枣4枚，调和营卫，以资巩固。

药后来信称：出汗明显减少，胃痛未作。

12月30日又来南京诊治。胃痛已除，形体较前为胖，饮食、二便正常。并于1978年1月2日再往鼓楼医院作胃镜检查，原萎缩性胃炎已消。病理报告：仅见胃体小弯重度浅表性胃炎，胃底小弯为轻度浅表性胃炎。嘱其间断服药，以冀巩固。

intermitently for consolidation.

2. Mr. Cai, male, 45.

History: The patient had stomachache for over 20 years that was aggravate during the past years. He usually took Vit U and probanthine. The gastroscopy by the Clinic Affliated to Provincial Council on June 5, 1976 revealed moderate chronic atrophic gastritis. The pathologic study in Drum-building Hospital showed moderate atrophic gastritis in lesser curvatrue of the antrum, the body and fundus.

The first visit: On May 31, 1976, the patient said that the stomachache lasted for over 20 years which was neglected at early stage and the illness progressed gradually. The patient had good appetite and constipation without acid reflux. Recently he had distension and pain in epigastrium and abdomen after meals with frequent belching and was sick of greasy food. The purplish tongue, thin white fur and thready wiry pulse were observed. The syndrome differentiation was middle insufficiency and qi-stagnation, and failure to descend stomach-qi. The treatment principle is to reinforce the middle and harmonize the stomach, regulate qi-flow and relieve pain.

Formula: Dangshen 9 g, Chaobaizhu 9 g, Chaodanggui 9 g, Hangbaishaoyao 9 g, Guizhi 6 g, Guangmuxiang

2. 蔡某,男,45 岁。

【病史】 胃痛已历 20 余年,常服维生素 U、普鲁本辛等,近一年来胃痛加重。1976 年 5 月 6 日在省委门诊部作胃镜检查,诊断为中度慢性萎缩性胃炎。鼓楼医院病理科报告:胃窦小弯、胃体小弯、胃底小弯—中度萎缩性胃炎。1976 年 5 月 31 日初诊:胃痛 20 余年,开始未予重视,以后病情逐渐加重,能食易饥,不泛酸,大便干结。近来食后则脘腹胀痛,频频嗳气,厌食油腻,舌质偏紫、苔薄白,脉弦细。中虚气滞,胃失和降,拟建中和胃,理气止痛。

党参 9 g,炒白术 9 g,炒当归9 g,杭白芍药 9 g,桂枝 6 g,广木香5 g,陈

5 g, Chenpi 6 g, Banxia 9 g, Zisugeng 5 g and Foshoupian 5 g.

The second visit: The stomach was relieved with less belching after 7 doses of the first formula. The distension in epigastrium still existed and low emotional status, thready wiry pulse and purplish tongue with thin white fur were observed. The syndrome differentiation was middle insufficiency, qi-stagnation, and phlegm stasis. Then Foshou was removed and Honghua was added instead. The symptoms were improved after 25 doses. The treatment was continued with pill for slow action.

Formula: Dangshen 50 g, Chaodanggui 50 g, Chaobaizhu 50 g, Guizhi 24 g, Hangbaishaoyao 50 g, Guangmuxiang 30 g, Banxia 50 g, Guangchenpi 24 g, Chaojianqu 60 g, Yunfuling 50 g, Zhigancao 15 g, Foshoupian 15 g, Chaozhike 50 g and Zhijineijin 50 g. These drugs were ground together and prepared into pills as big as size of semen firmianae with liquid decocted from Yuzhu 120 g and Dazao 240 g, taken 5 g once or twice a day.

The above formula had been taken for totally 4 months without attack of stomachache, abdominal distension, belching or constipation.

A gastroscopic check-up in Drum-building Hospital on Aug. 5, 1977 revealed chronic superficial gastritis.

皮 6 g,半夏 9 g,紫苏梗 5 g,佛手片 5 g。7 剂。

二诊:服药后,胃痛已止,嗳气亦少,胃脘仍作胀,精神差,面部赤脉如缕,脉弦细,苔薄白,质紫。中虚气滞,挟有痰瘀。原方去佛手,加红花 9 g。连服 25 剂后,症状续有改善,继予丸方缓图。

党参 50 g,炒当归 50 g,炒白术 50 g,桂枝 24 g,杭白芍药 50 g,广木香 30 g,半夏 50 g,广陈皮 24 g,炒建曲 60 g,云茯苓 50 g,炙甘草 15 g,佛手片 15 g,炒枳壳 50 g,炙鸡内金 50 g。

上药共研细末,另用玉竹 120 g、大枣 240 g 煎汤泛丸,如梧桐子大,每次服 5 g,每日 2 次。

上方共服 4 个月,胃痛未再作,腹胀消失,嗳气亦止,大便通畅。

1977 年 5 月 8 日去鼓楼医院胃镜复查,诊断为慢性浅表性胃炎。病

The pathologic report showed superficial gastritis in mucosa of antrum and lesser curvature. On Aug. 6, 1977, the patient had an attack of epigastric distension again, belching, thready wiry pulse and dark red tongue. The syndrome differentiation was middle insufficiency, qi-stagnation and indigestion. The symptoms disappeared after treated with the formula for regulating and reinforcing spleen.

Chapter Three   Experience from Professor He Hongbang

Section One   View on etiology and pathology

Professor He holds that this disorder belongs to gastric pain in TCM which is a common digestive disease. The treatment is relied on the analysis of the insufficiency or excess syndrome with focus on discrimination of similar disorders. The diseases could be divided into three types: insufficiency syndrome (including insufficiency cold, heat and insufficiency of both qi and yin), excessive syndrome (including qi-stagnation due to liver depressionand spleen insufficiency, heat stagnation due to stomach fire, injured stomach due to qi stagnation and phlegm stagnation with blood stasis) and integrated

理报告：胃窦小弯黏膜组织慢性炎变，胃体小弯为浅表性胃炎。患者于1977 年 6 月 8 日因食棒冰，自觉胃脘又作胀，嗳气不舒，脉弦细，舌质暗红。中虚气滞，运化不力。再用理气建中之剂调治，症状消失。

三、何宏邦教授治验

（一）对病因病机的认识

何教授认为本病属中医学胃脘痛范畴，为消化系统常见病、多发病，诊治本病，以虚实为纲，重视类证辨析，将本病概分三类证治。即虚证（包括虚寒证、虚热证、气阴两虚证）、实证（包括肝郁气滞证、胃火郁热证、气滞伤胃证、血瘀痰阻证）、虚实夹杂类（肝郁脾虚证）。其中以气阴两虚证在临床最为多见，占所观察两千余病例的三分之一以上；同时，无论何种证型多兼夹有或轻或重的血瘀证

慢性胃炎的中医特色疗法

excess and insufficiency (liver depression and spleen insufficiency. The type of insufficiency of both qi and yin is most common, being over one thirds of the cases observed. Meanwhile manifestion of blood stasis, mild or severe, can be found in any types and obvious symptoms of blood stasis in stomach vessels are usually seen when the disease lasting for long-term can enter the channel. So Professor He treated the disease with the emphasis on insufficiency of both qi and yin as well as blood stasis, and established Yangyin Yiqi Decoction and Danze Decoction by himself, which were respectively applied varyingly, showing satisfactory therapeutic effect.

Section Two   Experience and characteristics

In discussion of pathologic mechanism with insufficiency of both qi and yin, Professor He emphasizes on the yang nature of qi and yin nature of blood. This disease is due to insufficiency of stomach-yin originating form qi-consumption damaging yin. It initially attacks stomach and eventually affects spleen leading to insufficiency of middle qi, astringed middle yang, abnormality of digestion and then insufficiency of both qi and blood. The manifestation includes dull pain in epigstrium, relieved by pressing and eating, cold in the body and limbs as exterior symptoms while burning hot sensation in epigastrium

候,当本病发展到一定程度时,久病入络,临床往往出现以胃络血瘀积滞为主的显著症状。故何老将气阴两虚证和血瘀证作为诊治重点,针对两证病机自拟养阴益气汤与丹泽汤,分别随症加减施治于临床,效验颇著。

(二) 治疗经验与特色

何教授在有关本病气阴两虚的病理机制中,强调气为阳,血为阴,本证型应责之于胃阴不足,然其源则在气耗而阴伤。初病在胃,久病及脾,中气不足,中阳不展,致运化失常,气亏血少。临床症状见胃脘隐痛喜按,得食则缓,外有形寒肢冷,内则脘胀灼热,倦怠无力,寒热交错,口渴,小溲黄,舌胖质红,苔多剥脱,或舌前白苔、舌后浮黄,脉多虚弦。其治当以养阴益气为主,方用自拟养阴益气汤

and heartburn as interior symptoms, fatigue, intermittent chill and fever, thirst, yellow urine, red enlarged tongue with unfolliated tongue or white fur in the tip and floating yellow fur in the root, and weak wiry pulse. The treatment principle is mainly to nourish yin and reinforce qi and the formula Yangyin Yiqi decoction self-prescribed was applied varyingly according to symptoms.

Formula: Huangqi 20 g, Baishaoyao 20 g, Baihe 20 g, Shihu 15 g, Xiangyuan 15 g, Maimendong 15 g, Wuyao 10 g, Gancao 10 g, Huanglian 5 g, and Rougui 5 g. In case of qi-insufficiency, Buzhong Yiqi Decoction as qi tonics should be combined varyingly. In case of channel damage and blood stasis, Zelan 15 g and Muli 25 g are added; in case of dry and bitter mouth, Wumei 10 g and Longdanchao 7 g are added. The aim of this formula is to treat middle energizer for keeping its balanced function, and promote the physiological function of stomach and intestine. The key of spleen function and the key of stomach function are free passage, so in order to nourish the yin and body fluid, the first is to supplement the middle-qi and promote the transformation of Zhongzhou (middle energizer). Thus, medication should not only emphasize sweet herbs with cold nature to nourish stomach-yin and sweet herbs with sour nature to form yin and reinforce the stomach, but also avoid bitterness, dryness

随症加减。

【处方】 黄芪、白芍药、百合各20 g,石斛、香橼、麦门冬各15 g,乌药、甘草各10 g,黄连、肉桂各5 g。若偏气虚者合补中益气汤化裁;络损瘀结者,加泽兰15 g,牡蛎25 g;口干口苦重者加乌梅10 g,龙胆草7 g。本方乃根据"治中焦如衡",顺应脾胃的生理功能。脾贵健运,胃贵通顺,养阴津必先补益中气,以利中州转输之机。既重视甘寒滋养胃阴,甘酸化阴益胃,又避苦燥、阴腻之弊,以免困滞气机。

慢性胃炎的中医特色疗法

and yin greasiness to stagnate the activity of qi.

Section Three   Report of typical case

Mr. Yu, male, 53, the date of first visit: Oct. 27, 1982.

The patient had suffered pain in epigastrium and stomach for 20 years. It was aggravated in the past months. The patient had burning pain in the stomach and epigastrium, chill and shortness of breath, palpitation and oppression in the chest, overfatigue after exertion, dry and foul mouth, uneasiness after cold or hot meal, poor appetite and full distension, discomfort where pressed, swallowing acid and gastric upset, irregular stool, enlarged and dark tongue, floating white fur in the former part of the tongue and floating yellow fur in the root, deep, small and tight pulse, and a little larger pulse of Guan. The gastroscopy: atrophic gastritis. The syndrome differentation of TCM is insufficiency of both qi and yin. The treatment principle is to nourish the stomach-yin, supplement qi and harmonize the middle and formula of Yangyin Yiqi Decoction was used varyingly. The formula is Huangqi and Baihe, 20 g respectively, Dangshen, Danggui, Baishaoyao, Maimendong and Shihu, 15 g respectively; Wuyao, Wumei and Baidoukou, 10 g respectively; Rougui and Gancao, 5 g respectively.

（三）验案介绍

于某,男,53 岁,初诊:1982 年10 月 27 日。

患胃脘痛已 20 年,近月余加重,胃脘灼痛,畏冷短气,心悸胸闷,稍事劳作则疲惫不堪,口干且哕,饮食冷热均感不适,食少脘胀,按之不舒,吞酸嘈杂,大便欠调,舌胖质暗、苔前浮白后浮黄,脉沉小紧两关略大。胃镜检查,诊为"萎缩性胃炎",中医辨证属气阴两虚。治宜滋养胃阴,益气和中,投养阴益气汤化裁。

【处方】 黄芪、百合各 20 g,党参、当归、白芍药、麦门冬、石斛各 15 g,乌药、乌梅、白豆蔻各 10 g,肉桂、甘草各5 g。

随症加减用药 3 个月,诸症若失,胃镜复查为"胃窦部浅表性胃炎",余无异常。随访 1 年,胃痛未发。

After the formula had been used varyingly with the cond-
tions for three months, the symptoms disappeared and
gastroscopy check-up was superficial gastritis of the gastric antrum, whithout other abnormality. The stomachache didn't recur during one year of follow-up.

Chapter Four   Experience from Professor Zhao Jinduo

Section One   View on etiology and pathology

Professor Zhao holds that atrophic gastritis is
mainly characteristic of pain in the epigastrium and
stomach. Its pathology is complicated and often associ-
ated with liver (wood). Especially the onset is always
manifasted as liver-qi invading the stomach. The liver is
the organ of wind and wood which has the nature of or-
derly reaching. If the liver is damaged by depressed anger, the qi will be stagnated and crossed over to invade
the stomach (earth) of Yangming channel. Qi-stagnation for long-term tends to be transformed into fire
which tends to damage yin. Moreover, the long-term
disease can enter the channel which tends to cause stasis
and obstruction.

四、赵金铎教授治验

（一）对病因病机的认识

赵教授认为萎缩性胃炎以胃脘疼痛为主要临床表现，其病理变化复杂，多与肝木有关，尤其是发病之初，无不表现为肝木横逆犯胃之证。肝为风木之脏，性喜条达，若郁怒所伤则气滞横逆，侵犯阳明胃土而出现胃脘疼痛的症状。气郁久则易化火，化火则易伤阴。又久病入络，入络则易致瘀阻。

Section Two   Therapeutic exprience and characteristics

As to treatment principle of chronic atrophic gastritis, it is first important to sooth the liver and regulate the qi, to nourish the liver and save yin, and to activate liver blood and free its channels. The formula Jinlingzi Powder plus Yiguanjian Decoction is used varyingly. Chuanlianzi 10 g, Yanhusuo 3 g (taken as solution), Danggui 10 g, Gouqizi 6 g, Shashen 18 g, Maimendong 12 g, Shengdihuang 15 g, Foshoupian 9 g, Yujin 6 g and Guya and Maiya 15 g respectively. In case of insufficiency of stomach yin, proper amount of Shanyao is added; in case of insufficiency of liver-yin and stomach-yin, proper amount of Erzhi Pill to supplement yin. In case of obvious blood stasis, proper amont of Shixiaosan, Taoren, Chishaoyao and Danshen are added. Both the spleen and the stomach which correspond to middle energizer may fail to transform and digest food due to liver (wood) invading the stomach, resulting in declining of both qi and blood and viscera losing its nourishment. Therefore, in addition to pain in the epigastrium and stomach, a group of asthenic symptoms such as weight loss, fatigue, shortness of breath, dizziness, limp aching groin and knees, frequent urination, pale dark tongue, thin fur and fine weak pulse are observed. The spleen and stomach are the host and

（二）治疗经验与特色

对慢性萎缩性胃炎的治疗,赵教授主张首要注重疏肝理气,并注意养肝之体以济其阴,活肝之血以通其络。常用金铃子散合一贯煎加减出入为方：川楝子 10 g,延胡索粉 3 g（冲服）,当归 10 g,枸杞子 6 g,沙参 18 g,麦门冬 12 g,生地黄 15 g,佛手片 9 g,郁金 6 g,谷芽、麦芽各 15 g。胃阴虚者酌加山药,肝肾阴虚者可酌加二至丸以补阴,若瘀血明显,可酌加失笑散、桃仁、赤芍药、丹参等活血之品。脾胃均属中焦,因受肝木横逆之干扰而失运化之职,水谷不化,气血日衰,致使五脏六腑失之濡养。因而除胃脘痛外,常伴有消瘦、神疲、短气、头晕、腰膝酸软、小便频数、舌淡而暗、苔薄、脉细微无力等一系列虚劳见症。脾为肾之主,胃为肾之关,肾为先天,脾胃为后天,后天受阻,必然导致先天受害。肾失脾主之健运而致肾阴不足；水不涵木,肝木得以妄行。因此滋肾阴、强脾胃而济先后天,以制肝木之逆,是立法中不可忽

the gate of the kidney repectively. The kidney is of earlier heaven while the spleen and stomach are of later heaven. The later heaven is suffered which in turn damages the earlier heaven. The kidney loses its host of spleen to transport and transform which results in insufficiency of the kidney yin; the water fails to moisten wood which in turn liver (wood) takes advantage to stir abnormally. Therefore enriching kidney-yin and reinforcing spleen-stomach to aid both earlier and later heaven and then counteract liver-wood counterflow is an important step for the treatment principle. For this syndrome, Erzhi Pill (Double Supreme Pill) is added to main formula Yiguanjian Decoction to double the effect of supplementr the kidney, which is then combined with herbs of regulating liver and resoving depression such as Chenpi and Yujin, often causig the better result.

According to the clinical experience, eight to nine tenths of atropic gastritis is of yin-impairment pattern. Based on various damaged patterns of liver-yin, stomach-yin, spleen-yin, kidney-yin and their various degrees of damage, the treatment principle, prescription and medicines selection should be appropriate. In the course of treating the disease, the patients should be advised to regulate emotion and mind, control dieting and the living habits, only cooperated with the family to obtain good result.

视的环节。对此类见症，常在一贯煎的基础上加二至丸，以倍补肾之功，再配以陈皮、郁金等调肝解郁之品，往往能奏效。

临床体会，萎缩性胃炎阴伤者十之八九。根据伤肝阴、胃阴、脾阴、肾阴的不同，以及受害程度的深浅，在立法处方用药时务求恰如其分。在调治这类疾病的过程中，需嘱患者调情志、节饮食、慎起居，并需得到患者家属的密切配合，方可获效。

Section Three   Report of typical cases

Wu, female, 43 years old.

She had suffered from full distension in the stomach and epigastrium. Recently, she had attacks of pain, nausea after taking greasy and oily food and anorexia, with pale complexion, dizziness and blurred vision, fatigue and shortness of breath, fluster and palpitation, chill and cold in the limbs, no desire to drink despite thirst, urination after drinking water, frequent urination, pale tongue, thin white tongue fur deep, weak and rapid pulse. The diagnoses after examination at some hospital were "atrophic gastritis", "hypohydrochloria", "iron-defficiency anemia". The clinical syndrome differentiations were insufficiency of both kidney-yin and kidney-yang, and spleen losing transportation and transformation. Both the spleen and kidney should be strengthened, combined with medicine of rectifying Qi in treatment.

Nüzhenzi 15 g, Hanliancao 15 g, Gouqizi 12 g, Roucongrong 10 g, Danggui 12 g, Yuliren 9 g, Xiangyuanpi 12 g, Jineijin 6 g, Shanyao 20 g, Yuzhu 12 g, Shenggancao 6 g.

The second visit: After taking 7 doses of the medicine above-mentioned, the bowel movement became

（三）验案介绍

吴某某,女,43岁。

患胃脘闷堵胀满30年,近日来疼痛兼作,食油腻则欲吐,纳呆不食,伴见颜面苍白,头晕眼花,乏力短气,心慌心悸,畏寒肢冷,口干不欲饮,饮水即溲,小便频数,大便干结,舌质淡、苔薄白,脉沉微无力而数。经某医院检查确诊为"萎缩性胃炎"、"胃酸缺乏症"、"缺铁性贫血"。临床辨为肾阴阳两虚,脾失运化,治宜两固先后天,稍佐理气之品。

【处方】 女贞子15 g,旱莲草15 g,枸杞子12 g,肉苁蓉10 g,当归12 g,郁李仁9 g,香橼皮12 g,鸡内金6 g,山药20 g,玉竹12 g,生甘草6 g。

二诊:服上方7剂,大便通畅,脘腹胀满减轻。仍纳差,苔薄白舌淡、

free and full distension in the stomach and epigastrium
was relieved. However, there were still anorexia, pale
tongue, thin tongue fur with patch peeling in the middle,
and deep, weak and rapid pulse. The above-mentioned
formula was added with Baikouren and Houpohua.

The third visit: The patient's mental status became
better and other symptoms were improved. From the first
formula, Roucongrong and Yuliren were removed and
Danggui and Baishaoyao were added instead to regulate
and relieve all symptoms gradually. Then Liujunzi Decoction plus Liuwei Dihuang Pill were added with blood activating medicine to enhance the therapeutic effect. Having been treated for more than one year, the symptoms
disappared and the laboratory indicators related returned
to normal.

Chapter Five   Experience from Professor Yu Shangde

Section One   View on the etiology and pathology

Chronic gastritis with a long course is of insufficiency syndrome. Spleen-stomach insufficiency is considered
as the essential pathological changes of various chronic
gastritis. Chronic superficial gastritis is charact-eristic of

中见剥脱,脉沉微无力而数。前方佐入白蔻仁 5 g、厚朴花 9 g。

三诊:精神转佳,诸症均有好转,原方去肉苁蓉、郁李仁,加当归、白芍药调理,诸症渐平,后用六君子合六味地黄汤加活血药以善后。治疗年余,诸症渐退,复查时各种化验指标均无异常。

五、俞尚德教授治验

（一）对病因病机的认识

慢性胃炎有一个较长的病程,久病属"虚"。俞教授认为脾胃虚弱是各型慢性胃炎的基本病理变化。慢性浅表性胃炎以食欲减退、食后饱胀

the common symptoms such as anorexia, bloating and stomachache after meal, eructation (or acid reflux). Based on this syndrome differentiation, this disease is due to liver-stomach disharmony, especially liver depression and qi-stagnation. Therefore spleen-stomach is the pathological basis and liver depression and qi-stagnation is the pathomechanism in chronic superfial gastritis. According to the analysis of syndrome differentiation, there exist various degrees of blood dry and blood stasis. On the other hand, based on evolution characteristic of protracted disease entering the channel, the gastroscopic findings of superficial gastritis such as gastric mucosal congestion, redness, erosion, petechia are of local blood-dry and qi-stagnation, liver depression transforming into fire. Combined with white slimy fur and fine wiry pulse, chronic superficial gastritis is of insufficiency-cold reaction.

When the disease develops into atrophic gastritis, the course has been prolonged and the pathology has also been changed, in which spleen-stomach qi-insufficiency becomes prominent while liver-depression and qi-stagnation become the secondary so that the symptoms of liver-stomach disharmony is relieved while the manifestion of anerexia, loose stool and weight loss become more obvious, showing the symptoms of spleen-stomach qi-insufficiency. On the other hand, based on the differen-

作痛、嗳气（或有泛酸）等为较常见症状，据此辨证，一般是肝胃不和所致，并以肝郁气滞比较突出，故在慢性浅表性胃炎，脾胃气虚是病本，肝郁气滞为主要病机。审病辨证分析，各型胃炎还都存在着不同程度的血涩或血瘀的情况，另一方面从久病入络的演变规律认证，并结合胃镜检查所见，如：浅表性胃炎可见黏膜充血、潮红、糜烂、出血点等，为局部血涩气滞，肝郁化火的征象。再参以慢性浅表性胃炎患者的苔多白滑，脉多细弦看，亦为虚寒反应。

当病变演进至萎缩性胃炎时，则历时更久，病机亦有转化，脾胃气虚更为突出，肝郁气滞变为次要环节，故相应的一般肝胃不和症状反而减轻，而食欲不振、大便不实、体重减轻等表现较为明显，愈加显示出脾胃气虚的症状。另一方面从久病入络的演变规律认证，并结合胃镜检查所见，萎缩性胃炎见黏膜苍白、菲薄、蓝

tiation analysis of protracted disease entering the channel, the gastropic findings of superficial gastritis such as pale and thin gastric mucosa as well as veins observed are due to local blood-stasis and obstructing-channel, and insuficient qi-blood movement. Moreover fine and wiry pulse of patients with atrophic gastritis is of insufficiency-cold syndrome. To sum up, for both chronic superfial gastritis and atrophic gastritis, is more than stomach-Yin insufficinecy and insufficiency-cols syndrome clinically.

Section Two   Therapeutic experience and characteristics

Nourishing the stomach and harmonizing the center as well as soothing the liver and regulating qi are the treatment principle for the chronic suerficial gastritis. The formula used is "Superfical Gastritis Formula": Huangqi 10 – 15 g, Chaobaizhu 10 – 15 g, (or Guizhi 10 g), Gancao 10 – 15 g, Chishaoyao 10 – 15 g, Danggui 10 g, Jiuyanhusuo 10 g, Foshougan (or Chenxiangyuan) 10 g, Baijiangcao 15 – 30 g, Baihuasheshecao (or Pugongying, or Banzhilian) 15 – 30 g, Chaozhike (or Chuanhoupo) 10 g, (note: Fuling 15 – 30 g had better be added if Gancao amount of each dose is over 12 g). In case of gastric mucosa erosion, Dangshen 15 g, Shengbaiji 6 g and Zhiruxiang 3 g, Shensanqi 3 g; in case of qi-stagnation

色血管透见等,为局部血瘀阻络,气血运营不足所致。而且萎缩性胃炎舌苔多白滑,脉多细弦,亦为虚寒反应。总之,无论是慢性浅表性胃炎,还是慢性萎缩性胃炎,临床上胃阴不足证少有,而虚寒证多见。

(二)治疗经验与特色

慢性浅表性胃炎治疗时以养胃和中、疏肝理气兼活血为主要治疗大法,采用处方浅表性胃炎方:黄芪10～15 g,炒苍术 10～15 g,(或桂枝10 g),甘草(炙或生)10～15 g,赤芍药 10～15 g,当归 10 g,酒延胡索10 g,佛手柑(或陈香橼)10 g,败酱草15～30 g,白花蛇舌草(或蒲公英、半枝莲)15～30 g,炒枳壳(或川厚朴)10 g(注:甘草用量每剂在 12 g 以上时宜加茯苓 15～30 g)。伴有胃黏膜糜烂者,加党参 15 g,生白及 6 g,制乳香3 g,参三七 3 g 等;气滞饱胀者,

and full distension, Xiangfu 10 g, Jinlingzi 10 g, Chenxiang
qu 20 g; in case of gastric upset, Dangshen 15 g and Zhiyuzhu
30 g are added; in case of acid reflux, Danwuzhuyu 4 g and
Bichengqie 10 g are added; in case of more regurgitationg of
digestive fluids; Sumu 10 g (with Zhike), Zhibanxia 10 g and
Daizheshi 30 g are added.

The therapy for chronic atrophic gastritis is to supplement the middle and boost qi as well as free the channel and removing stasis. The Formula for Atropic Gastritis was made by Professor Yu: Zhihuangqi 10 -30 g, Dangshen 15 -20 g, Zhigancao 15 - 20 g, Baishaoyao
30 - 50 g, Guizhi 6 - 10 g, Danggui 10 g, Ezhu 10 g, Honghua 5 g (or Sanqi powder 3 g divided and swallowed),
Baihuasheshecao (or Qiyeyizhihua or Baijiangcao)
10 - 20 g and Fuling 30 g are added. Professor Yu further-
ly indicated that chronic gastritis has multiple clinical
manifestations which seem not all due to inflammation
process. So its treatment could be only aimed at improving clinical symptoms not at changing the pathological
changes of inflammation; moreover the occurence of
both superficial and atrophic gastritis in different part of
the stomach is not rare and then the treatment should
consider both clinical manifestations and degree of inflammation and atrophy in order to modify the formula.

用香附 10 g,金铃子 10 g,沉香曲 20 g
等;嘈杂者,用党参 15 g,制玉竹 30 g
等;泛酸者用淡吴茱萸 4 g,荜澄茄
10 g等;消化液反流多者,用苏木 10 g
(配枳壳),制半夏 10 g,代赭石
30 g 等。

慢性萎缩性胃炎治疗宜补中益
气,通络行瘀为主。处方为自拟萎缩
性胃炎方:炙黄芪 10～30 g,党参
15～20 g,炙甘草 15～20 g,白芍药
30～50 g,桂枝 6～10 g,当归 10 g,莪
术 10 g,红花 5 g(或以三七粉 3 g分
吞),白花蛇舌草(或七叶一枝花或败
酱草)10～20 g,茯苓30 g。俞教授进
一步指出:慢性萎缩性胃炎临床表现
复杂多样,似乎并非全是由于炎症过
程引起的,所以其治疗既不能仅以临
床症状改善为目的,也不可只着意于
病理组织学"炎症"的改变;再则慢性
胃炎患者,在胃的不同部位发生浅表
性与萎缩性病变并存者为数不鲜,治
疗时应结合临床症状并视浅表炎症
与萎缩的程度孰轻孰重,加减处方
用药。

Section Three   Report of typical cases

1. Qin, male, 50. The date of first visit: April 18, 1979.

Gastroscopy in April 1979: Congestion in gastric body with plenty of white mucous plaque; local mucosal erosion in greater curvature; congestion in gastric angle; rough mocosa in gastric antrum with profuse muocus plaque; rough mucosa in front wall of gastric antrum, showing polypoid projection; reflux of digestive fluids. Diagnosis: chronic superficial gastritis accompanied by local erosion. The complaint at the first visit: There was abdominal pain in the epigastrium accompanied by melena and bloody stool, with frequent attacks of bleeding in June, December and March 1978. Recently there appeared epigastrium pain, fullness after eating more, eructation, patch peeling in the middle tongue, thin, white and slimy fur, and fine slimy pulse. Prescription: The Formular of Superficial Gastritis, added with Dangshen 10 g, Maimendong 10 g, Shensanqi 3 g, Qingdai 3 g, and Zhike removed. After taking medicine for two weeks, the symptoms disappeared. After 10 weeks, his tongue fur had no patch peeling, the pusle became fine and wiry. The course lasted for 13 weeks in total.

Gastroscopy in July of 1979: a littel mucous plaque at

（三）验案介绍

1. 秦某,男,50 岁。初诊:1979 年 4 月 18 日。

1979 年 4 月胃镜检查:胃体充血,附多量白色黏液斑;大弯侧黏膜局限性糜烂;胃角充血;胃窦部黏膜增粗,附多量黏液斑;幽门前壁黏膜增粗,呈息肉样隆起。有消化液反流。诊断:慢性浅表性胃炎伴局限性糜烂。初诊时诉:1978 年 5 月,有上腹部痛伴黑便出血,以后于同年 6 月、12 月及今年 3 月有反复出血。近时上腹痛,多食作胀,嗳气,舌中剥、苔薄白滑,脉细滑。处方:浅表性胃炎方加党参 10 g,麦门冬 10 g,参三七 3 g,青黛 3 g 等,去枳壳。服药 2 周,症状消失。治疗 10 周,舌已不剥,脉转细弦。共服药 13 周。

1979 年 7 月胃镜复查:胃体大

慢性胃炎的中医特色疗法

greater or lesser curvature, white and red colour in mucosa, little prominance 2 cm apart from the pyloric opening, edema, smooth surface with congestion. Diagnosis: superficial gastritis. Then Sanqi powder was removed, taking medicine intermittenly for 17 weeks, and checked again, showing that slight white and red colour in gastric body, white and red in the pylolus, a little rough mucosa, much mucous plaque. Rougher mucosa in front wall of antrum with polypoid prominence. The diagnosis was superficial gastritis.

2. Yu, male, 26 years old. The date of the first visit: October 23, 1995.

The gastroscopy of November of 1995: Congestion in cardia and fundus, scattered bleeding spot in submucosa of angular region of the body: Congestion in the stomach angle and bleeding spot in the plexiform mucosa of the upper and lower border; congestion and edema in the antrum, bleeding spot and focal erosion; loose pylorus. The diagnosis was chronic superficial erosive gastritis. The pathogenesis: antrum chronic severe superficial-atrophic gastritis (active) accompanied by severe intestinal metaplasia, lymphatic follicle formed. HP postive (strong). The intestine fluids dyed were mainly complete intestinal and colonic metaplasia and minorly was incomplete intestinal metaplasia. At the first visit, the patient

小弯黏液斑少许,黏膜红白相间,无糜烂。胃窦部有黏液斑,黏膜红白相间。小弯侧距幽门孔 2 cm 处稍隆起,水肿,表面光滑,无充血。诊断:浅表性胃炎。以后除去三七粉,断续服药 17 周,再作胃镜复查:胃体轻度红白相间。胃窦部红白相间,黏膜稍粗,黏液斑多。幽门前壁黏膜增粗,呈息肉样隆起。诊断:浅表性胃炎。

2. 余某,男,26 岁。初诊:1995年 10 月 23 日。

1995 年 11 月胃镜检查:贲门、胃底充血,胃体垂直部有散在黏膜下出血斑点;胃角充血,上下缘有丛状黏膜下出血斑点;胃窦充血水肿,有黏膜下出血斑点及灶性糜烂;幽门松弛。诊断:慢性浅表糜烂性胃炎。病理:(胃窦)慢性重度浅表-萎缩性胃炎(活动期)伴重度肠化,淋巴滤泡形成。HP 强阳性。黏液染色肠化以完全性小肠型和结肠型为主,少数不完全性小肠型。初诊时诉胃病史 6 年,胃脘胀痛,嘈杂,微灼热感,有嗳气,不泛酸,纳便正常。舌质偏红少苔,

complained that he had had stomach disease for 6 years, distension and pain in the stomach and epigastrium, gastric upset, slight heartburn, eructation, no acid reflux and normal stool, reddish tongue with less fur, and wiry slow pulse. He had heavy smoking and drinking and was advised to give them up. Prescription: The Formula of Atrophic Gastritis. The ingredients were Zhihuangqi 10 - 30 g, Dangshen 15 - 20 g, Zhigancao 15 - 20 g, Baishaoyao 30 - 50 g, Guizhi 6 -10 g, Danggui 10 g, Ezhu 10 g, Honghua 5 g (or Sanqi powder 3 g divided and swallowed), Baihuasheshecao (or Qiyeyizhihua or Baijiangcao) 10 - 20 g, Fuling 30 g. Because of erosion and bleeding in the stomach mucosa, red tongue and wiry pulse, Guizhi was removed and Baiji 6 g, Ruxiang 3 g, Baijiangcao 20 g were added. After taking the medicine for 4 weeks, the symptoms disappered with clear fur and a little wiry pulse. The patient was continued with the original formula, for 12 weeks in total.

Gastroscopy of February 4, 1996: Congestion in cardia and the body, severe congestion and edema in stomach angle, congestion and edema in pylolus with much secretion and scattered bleeding spot. The pylolous was loose, and there were congestion and edema in the borders. Diagnosis: Middle superficial gastritis. Pathogenesis: (antrum) Chronic superficial gastritis. HP (-).

脉较弦缓。有酷嗜烟酒恶习,嘱戒烟酒。处方:萎缩性胃炎方,炙黄芪10～30 g,党参15～20 g,炙甘草15～20 g,白芍药30～50 g,桂枝6～10 g,当归10 g,莪术10 g,红花5 g(或以三七粉3 g分吞),白花蛇舌草(或七叶一枝花或败酱草)10～20 g,茯苓30 g。鉴于有胃黏膜糜烂与出血,舌质较红,脉象较弦,故减去桂枝,加白及6 g,乳香3 g,败酱草20 g。服药4周后症状消失,舌净,脉微弦,续服原方,共服药12周。

1996年2月4日胃镜复查:贲门充血,胃体充血,胃角充血水肿明显,胃窦充血水肿,分泌物多,有个别黏膜下出血点。幽门较松弛,边缘充血水肿。诊断:中度浅表性胃炎。病理:(胃窦)慢性中度浅表性胃炎。HP(一)。

Index

索 引

慢性胃炎的中医特色疗法

An English-Chinese Guide to Clinical Treatment of Common Diseases

Typical TCM Therapy for Viral Hepatitis

Typical TCM Therapy for Primary Glomerulonephritis

Typical TCM Therapy for Chronic Gastritis

Typical TCM Therapy for Lung Cancer

Typical TCM Therapy for Bronchial Asthma

Typical TCM Therapy for Diabetes

Typical TCM Therapy for Primary Hypertension

Typical TCM Therapy for Rheumatoid Arthritis

Typical TCM Therapy for Cervical Spondylosis

Typical TCM Therapy for Cholelithiasis

（英汉对照）常见病临证要览

病毒性肝炎的中医特色疗法

原发性肾小球肾炎的中医特色疗法

慢性胃炎的中医特色疗法

肺癌的中医特色疗法

支气管哮喘的中医特色疗法

糖尿病的中医特色疗法

高血压病的中医特色疗法

类风湿关节炎的中医特色疗法

颈椎病的中医特色疗法

胆石症的中医特色疗法